Macroevolutionary Dynamics

Macroevolutionary Dynamics

Species, Niches, and Adaptive Peaks

NILES ELDREDGE

*The American Museum
of Natural History*

McGraw-Hill Publishing Company

New York   St. Louis   San Francisco   Auckland
Bogotá   Hamburg   London   Madrid   Milan   Mexico
Montreal   New Delhi   Panama   Paris   São Paulo
Singapore   Sydney   Tokyo   Toronto

Library of Congress Cataloging-in-Publication Data

Eldredge, Niles.
 Macroevolutionary dynamics.

 Bibliography: p.
 Includes index.
 1. Evolution. I. Title
 QH366.2.E52 1989 575   88-32585
 ISBN 0-07-019474-2

1234567890   DOCDOC   8965432109

ISBN 0-07-019474-2

ISBN 0-07-019476-9 {PBK.}

The editors for this book were Jennifer Mitchell and Su-
san Thomas, the designer was Naomi Auerbach, and the
production supervisor was Suzanne W. Babeuf. It was
set in Century Schoolbook by the McGraw-Hill Publishing Company, Professional & Reference Division Composition Unit.

Printed and bound by R. R. Donnelley & Sons Company.

*For more information about other McGraw-Hill materi-
als, call 1-800-2-MCGRAW in the United States. In other
countries, call your nearest McGraw-Hill office.*

Contents

Preface

It is time (as an esteemed colleague recently remarked) to confront once again the fact that polar bears are white. To some extent, attention has been diverted over the past 20 years from the traditional Darwinian focus on adaptive transformation of the phenotypic properties of organisms through natural selection. In these years, evolutionary theory has been enriched by a host of ideas on additional causal elements contributing to the history of life, from molecular processes at the genic and developmental levels up through notions of group and species selection at the higher levels.

Though adaptation itself has been somewhat eclipsed through all this, it has certainly not been without its vigorous defenders as well. Indeed, adaptation remains the central theme of theoretical evolutionary biology. And yet we still do not know very much more about the nature of the processes underlying the stasis and change of phenotypic features than Darwin himself was able to specify. We do know more, of course, about the workings of inheritance and the source of genetic novelty, and even something about the functional connection between genetic information and the development of organismic phenotypes.

But we have rather little theory as yet that tells us under what circumstances we are to expect adaptive change. When does adaptive change occur in evolution? What determines the stasis so commonly observed throughout the histories of most species? What factors govern the degree of adaptive change when it does occur? It is the evolutionary context of adaptive change that concerns me most in this book. I think it is entirely possible to formulate theory that addresses these issues, and I have attempted to do so as the prime goal of this book.

Macroevolution, however it is precisely defined, always connotes "large-scale phenotypic evolutionary change." As I will detail in Chap. 1, there are theories of molecular and developmental processes that explore the possibility of significant evolutionary change at those levels. The focus of this book, in contrast, is on the organismic and higher levels—populations, species, monophyletic taxa, and local and regional ecosystems. And, just as there are theories of macroevolutionary processes at lower levels, there are higher-level evolutionary processes that may result in the accrual of little or no significant phenotypic change, a fact which violates the commonplace understanding of "macroevolution." This book addresses all degrees of adaptive organismic phenotypic change, viewed especially from the biotic perspective (i.e., with the understanding that organisms are parts of larger-scale biological entities, such as species or ecosystems).

I write this book for fellow professionals at all stages of development. Today's students will be the ones to decide which lines of thought from past and present generations will be worth pursuing. Veterans who have been at the wars for some time might find the first two chapters or so a bit slow, if only because the material (especially in Chap. 2) will be so familiar to them. But the research paradigm of adaptation as practiced under the synthesis, while still very much alive today, may not be as familiar to younger members of the evolutionary biology profession as it is to us older practitioners; it deserves careful consideration, which I have endeavored to provide in Chap. 2, before Chap. 3 begins the analysis and extension of more recent developments.

My aim is to probe and to build, not merely to recite. My own views have undergone a change (nothing drastic) over the past 20 years; there is still much to be learned. May the efforts here stimulate others to push back the curtains shrouding the mysteries of evolution still further.

Niles Eldredge

Acknowledgment

I am grateful to Dr. Marjorie Grene
for careful review of an earlier draft
of this book. I also thank
Dr. E. C. Olson for
reviewing the manuscript.

Credits

The author is grateful for permission to reprint material from the following sources:

Walter J. Bock, *Bulletin of the Carnegie Museum of Natural History*, vol. 13. Copyright © 1979. By permission.

Theodosius Dobzhansky, *Genetics and the Origin of Species.* Copyright © 1937, 1951, Columbia University Press. By permission.

Niles Eldredge, *Annual Review of Ecology and Systematics*, vol. 17. Copyright © 1986 by Annual Reviews Inc. By permission.

Niles Eldredge and Joel Cracraft, *Phylogenetic Patterns and the Evolutionary Process.* Copyright © 1980, Columbia University Press. By permission.

Philip D. Gingerich, *American Journal of Science*, vol. 276. Copyright © 1976. By permission.

David L. Hull, *Annual Review of Ecology and Systematics*, vol. 11, Copyright © 1980 by Annual Reviews, Inc. By permission.

William Miller III, *Lethaia*, vol. 19. Copyright © 1986. By permission.

J. E. Morton, *Molluscs.* Copyright © 1958, Hutchinson and Company, London.

C. M. Newman et al., *Nature*, vol. 315. Copyright © 1985, Macmillan Magazines Ltd. By permission.

S. A. Schaefer and G. V. Lauder, *Systematic Zoology*, vol. 35. Copyright © 1986. By permission.

George G. Simpson, *Tempo and Mode in Evolution.* Copyright © 1944, Columbia University Press. By permission.

Steven M. Stanley, *Proceedings of the National Academy of Science*, vol. 72. Copyright © 1975. By permission.

Steven M. Stanley, *Paleobiology*, vol. 11, Copyright © 1985. By permission.

Macroevolution: Some Basic Considerations

Evolution is the proposition that all organisms on earth, past, present, and future, are descended from a common ancestor that lived at least 3.5 billion years ago, the age of the oldest fossil bacteria yet reliably identified. Darwin (1859), saving the word "evolved" for his last sentence, used the phrase "descent with modification" for the biological phenomenon we call "evolution" today. In his only diagram in *On the Origin of Species*, Darwin depicted the results of his process of "descent with modification" as a historical, branching pattern. New branches arise from old; from time to time, innovations are developed (largely via his proposed mechanism of natural selection) and are passed along to descendants. The pattern of branching and modification, Darwin saw, automatically leads to another sort of pattern, in which the similarities of organisms are nested in a complex fashion. A hierarchical array of evolutionary novelties—*homologies*—automatically results from the simple process of branching and descent with modification. This pattern, in fact, is the most important prediction about the way the biological world is structured that arises from the scientific hypothesis of "evolution."

If we view biological history and its underlying processes in Darwin's original fashion, there is little need to distinguish micro- from macroevolution. Evolution in general is simply biological history. Darwin was very much a uniformitarian: accordingly, the processes observable in biological systems today are assumed to have been at work in the past. And, especially, those processes observed to cause small, incremental changes within the temporal scale of human observation may confidently be expected to accumulate into truly large-scale changes as vastly longer increments of time pass by. Thus, to Darwin, there was no difference in principle between the nature or kind of change that may accrue within any segment of the tree of life over a short interval and the kind that may accrue over a much longer period of time. Only the amount of evolutionary change, as a more or less direct function of elapsed time, could distinguish between small- and large-scale evolution—i.e., microevolution vs. macroevolution.

But what, exactly, "evolves" in evolution? The pat answer is "species." Yet, as we shall see in later chapters, in some conceptualizations of the nature of species, it is as difficult to imagine species evolving as it is to maintain that organisms evolve. Again, turning to Darwin's original formulation clarifies the matter considerably, providing a good starting point for exploring the matter further. To Darwin, the original problem demanding explanation—the entire raison d'être of evolutionary theory—is the fact of organic design in nature. Before Darwin, the standard explanation of design in nature, the apparently meticulous fit of organisms into their worldly surroundings, invoked a supernatural Creator. Creationists today still call on William Paley's watchmaker: just as a complex instrument such as a watch implies an intelligent watchmaker underlying its construction, so too do intricately structured organisms bespeak the handiwork of an intelligent Creator. Darwin countered this age-old explanation of organic design with the mindless, materialistic, and thoroughly naturalistic process of natural selection, thus neatly placing the problem of organic design squarely within the realm of biological science. We will return to natural selection, its nature and role in the evolutionary process, in later chapters. The point to be stressed here is that Darwin developed his theory of evolution through natural selection to explain the distribution of organismic traits in the Recent biota, and by extension, throughout the entire history of life. To Darwin, it was these traits (what we now call the *phenotypic features* or *properties* of organisms) that evolve. Through time, traits either stay the same or become modified—the literal meaning of "descent with modification."

Darwin, though ignorant of the principles of heredity, of course knew that organisms tend to resemble their parents, just as animal and plant breeders have observed presumably from Neolithic times, some 10,000 years ago. With the advent and rapid growth of genetics in the early years of the twentieth century, some biologists began equating evolution not just with the explanation of phenotypic diversity but with the genetic factors underlying the phenotypic traits. Thus, from the mid-1930s on (as the modern synthesis developed and became the dominant evolutionary theory over the past 50 years), evolution was most commonly defined as "change in gene content and frequency within a population" (as in Dobzhansky, 1951, p. 16: "Evolution is a change in the genetic composition of populations").

If we follow Darwin's lead and speak of the evolution not of *entities* (such as organisms, populations,[1] species, or monophyletic taxa) but of *traits*, we converge on a visualization of evolution as the maintenance and modification of genetically based information—the most general sense of "evolution" as used in this book. And thus we can retain the distinction between micro- and macroevolution as simply a matter of scale: macroevolution is genetic change accumulated over the vast periods of time associated with the geological history of life on earth. As a first approximation, this definition, in accord with the thinking of a majority of evolutionary biologists, will suffice. As we delve more deeply into macroevolutionary theory, however, the situation becomes far more complex.

Attitudes Toward Macroevolution

Darwin's view—that all evolution is essentially a function of adaptive change under the predominant control of natural selection—forms the basis of the modern view of evolution under the *evolutionary synthesis*.[2] The advent of genetics, the fledgling science of heredity, with the rediscovery of Mendel's "laws" at the beginning of the twentieth century contributed to a partial eclipse of the Darwinian approach to evolution and "natural history." It was simply assumed by many biologists around the turn of the century that an understanding of the physiological mechanisms of heredity, including the principles underlying change in the genetic materials, would suffice to explain evolution. An early example comes from the work of Hugo De Vries, one of the three biologists to independently rediscover Mendel's work. De Vries observed sudden, large-scale phenotypic changes in his experimental plants of the evening primrose *Oenothera*, leading him to postulate an internal mechanism for the origin of new species. De Vries was joined by many other biologists of his time, understandably enamored with new technologies for probing the inner (including intracellular) chemical and physical workings of organisms. Yet, as some molecular biologists of the present time realize, understanding evolution to be maintenance and modification of genetically based information by no means implies that the dynamics of the evolutionary process are to be understood solely with reference to the physicochemical structure and processes of the genome.

Yet the fast-growing science of genetics was not the only source of disarray for the Darwinian view of the evolutionary process. Paleontologists, at least since the time of the American Edward Drinker Cope, were fond of espousing internal, "vitalistic" factors as evolutionary mechanisms. Paleontologists have had an abiding interest in long-term evolutionary trends that struck Cope and many others as linear or "rectilinear." "Orthogenesis," a term coined by Haacke (1893; *fide* Simpson, 1944), describes a pattern of linear directional change in phylogeny, a pattern generally thought in presynthesis days to reflect internal evolutionary processes. This line of thinking, at least in paleontological circles, reached its culmination in the work of vertebrate paleontologist Henry Fairfield Osborn, whose theory of orthogenesis (later called "aristogenesis") saw linear evolutionary change as the result of directed mechanisms of genetic change arising from within organisms themselves, a mechanism, moreover, taking precedence over natural selection if not supplanting it altogether.

Although there is still plenty of controversy within evolutionary theory, the advent of the synthesis at least marked the end of an era when specialists in disparate disciplines could safely ignore one another. In the 1920s it was still possible for a paleontologist such as Osborn, if he did not like the available theories offered by the geneticists of his day, to invent his own theory of genetics, basically out of whole cloth, but fashioned in such a way as seemed to fit his own interpretation of the data of the fossil record more satisfactorily. The synthesis, though it now seems to some biologists rather less of a true synthesis than it was at first purported to be (see Gould, 1980*a;* Eldredge, 1985*a;* Brooks and Wiley, 1986), was a consensus statement written by geneticists of several sorts (including what would now be called theoretical population geneticists, experimentalists, and field naturalists), systematists, and paleontologists. The basic tenets of the synthesis were accepted by a majority of working biologists. Though communication between these disparate fields has remained at times rather tenuous, there is considerably more caution displayed when a practitioner of one discipline discusses areas that fall under the purview of another discipline. Sometimes the communication, and even cooperation, is far better than simple acknowledgment that other approaches to understanding evolution exist. For this we must thank the early architects of the evolutionary synthesis.

Most of the seeming inconsistencies between the early findings of genetics and the Darwinian view of evolutionary processes were reconciled in the 1920s and early 1930s. Mutations, at first commonly thought to be invariably large-scale and usually harmful in their phenotypic expression (because such mutations are simply the easiest to observe, and the phenotype was the only means of studying the genotype until the structure of DNA and RNA was elucidated in the 1950s), lately came to be seen as the ultimate source of new variation. The work of three geneticists in particular—Ronald Fisher and J. B. S. Haldane in England and the American Sewall Wright—marks a distinct and powerful return to Darwinian processes (though Wright is perhaps best known for his advocacy of the "shifting balance theory" and "genetic drift," a theoretical outlook that sees random processes in addition to natural selection as important in effecting genetic change in the evolutionary process). Fisher, in particular, virtually equated "evolution" with "adaptive change through natural selection." These three geneticists effectively set the stage for the first, and arguably most important, formulation of the synthesis, the first edition of Theodosius Dobzhansky's (1937a) *Genetics and the Origin of Species.*

Dobzhansky's book effectively sets forth the basis of the modern theory of evolution. At the same time, it represents a return to the Darwinian vision of adaptation through natural selection as the cornerstone of the evolutionary process. Dobzhansky was especially concerned to integrate theoretical and practical laboratory results of geneticists with observations he and others had made in the field. Repeatedly, Dobzhansky (1937a) stresses that theoretical and even experimental work is of limited value if it cannot be extended rigorously to an understanding of observations made in the wild. And herein lies a clue to understanding Dobzhansky's attitude on macroevolution, an attitude which very much echoed Darwin's own ideas on long-term evolutionary change but which is based as well on strong epistemological[3] considerations. Dobzhansky wrote (1937a, p. 12):

> We are compelled at the present level of knowledge reluctantly to put a sign of equality between the mechanisms of micro- and macro-evolution, and, proceeding on this assumption, to push our investigations as far ahead as this working hypothesis will permit.

As we shall see in the immediately ensuing chapters, Dobzhansky proceeded to fashion a theory that indeed saw macroevolution as the accumulation of microevolutionary changes over periods of time extending far beyond human capacity for direct experimentation and observation. The point to stress here is the methodological consideration that led Dobzhansky to this view. Seeing evolution as modification of the genetic composition of populations through time, Dobzhansky reasoned that enough change could be observed experimentally and in the wild to establish the general principles governing such change. These are the "evolutionary dynamics," as he called them, processes working at the population level that use the raw materials afforded by "evolutionary statics," which are the physiological processes of inheritance—including mutation, the ultimate source of genetic variation. *If,* Dobzhansky reasoned, there are long-term processes arising from or affecting the genetic constitution of organisms or populations that differ from those processes observable in modern-

day organisms over the short spans of time afforded to human observation, then we are likely to remain in ignorance of them. That is why
Dobzhansky wrote that "we are compelled...reluctantly" to equate
macro- with microevolution. Microevolution is all we can study scientifically.

In writing that brief statement on macroevolution, Dobzhansky
firmly rooted evolutionary biology in general within the realm of empirical science. We simply must assume that genetic processes and entities as understood in living organisms are characteristic in the main
of processes and entities that occurred in organisms throughout the
approximately 3.5 billion years of organic history on earth. Nor does it
make sound sense epistemologically to insist upon unknown (and perhaps in principle even unknowable) genetic mechanisms to explain
large-scale patterns in the evolutionary history of life. That some authors have recently maintained that macroevolution cannot be understood strictly as an outgrowth of organismic and population-level processes of genetic change hinges on ontological issues, specifically the
claim that species and monophyletic taxa are themselves large-scale
entities; I return to a discussion of this viewpoint immediately below,
in this chapter.

Thus, ever since Dobzhansky's important book, all serious students
of the evolutionary process have agreed that whatever is said about
the nature of the evolutionary process must at least be consistent with
what is thought to be established concerning the principles of heredity, the origin of variation, and the nature of random (drift) and deterministic (natural selection) processes governing gene content and
frequency within natural populations. Paleontologist George Gaylord
Simpson was particularly eloquent on the need for such consistency as
he sought (in his 1944 *Tempo and Mode in Evolution*) to reconcile the
principles of genetics with the data of paleontology. In an amusing
characterization of the relation between genetics and paleontology
just before the advent of the synthesis, Simpson wrote (1944, p. xv):

> Not long ago paleontologists felt that a geneticist was a person who shut
> himself in a room, pulled down the shades, watched small flies disporting
> themselves in milk bottles, and thought that he was studying nature. A
> pursuit so removed from the realities of life, they said, had no signifi-
> cance for the true biologist. On the other hand, the geneticists said that
> paleontology had no further contributions to make to biology, that its
> only point had been the completed demonstration of the truth of evolu-
> tion, and that it was a subject too purely descriptive to merit the name
> "science." The paleontologist, they believed, is like a man who under-
> takes to study the principles of the internal combustion engine by stand-
> ing on a street corner and watching the motor cars whizz by.

Then Simpson posed an intriguing proposition: If it is indeed true (and, as we have seen, as Dobzhansky had already claimed) that the "statics" and "dynamics" of the evolutionary process lie squarely within the province of genetics, nonetheless the large-scale patterns in the history of life are full of evolutionary implications. Specifically, Simpson argued that only someone well versed in historical patterns would be able to determine what are the specific *combinations* of "evolutionary determinants" (Simpson's general term for genetic factors important in evolution, e.g., mutation rate, natural selection, etc.). Simpson wrote (1944, p. xvii):

> ...experimental biology in general and genetics in particular have the grave defect that they cannot reproduce the vast and complex horizontal extent of the natural environment and, particularly, the immense span of time in which population changes really occur. They may reveal what happens to a hundred rats in the course of ten years under fixed and simple conditions, but not what happened to a billion rats in the course of ten million years under the fluctuating conditions of earth history. Obviously, the latter problem is much more important.

Thus Simpson set out to use known genetic factors in particular combinations to explain large-scale patterns in the history of life. Though one might criticize both his characterization and his explanation of such patterns, in spirit his approach is particularly valuable in the investigation of the relation between large-scale evolutionary patterns and the underlying processes that have produced them. Simpson agreed with Dobzhansky not only in the uniformitarian assumption that genetic entities and processes known to exist and operate currently are the same as those characteristic of organisms of the past, but that such genetic mechanisms are also sufficient to yield a complete understanding of evolutionary change. Yet insight into how those genetic entities, processes, and parameters combine to yield characteristic patterns in the history of life is not likely to spring solely from a consideration of single populations, whether in the laboratory or even observed in the wild. Time and numbers of organisms are likely to be important factors, as Simpson said. And, as we shall see in later chapters, the roles played by large-scale biological systems now appear critical as well to a more thorough understanding of the evolutionary process.

"Functional" and "Historical" Science

Dobzhansky's epistemological formulation—in which evolutionary mechanisms are studied in the laboratory and the field on living organisms and assumed to produce large-scale effects over long periods of time—is logical and appealing. As a corollary, some biologists, such as systematist Ernst Mayr and paleontologist G. G. Simpson, have emphasized a distinction between two *kinds* of science, "functional" and "historical" science, which are said to differ in their inherent subject matter and, most importantly, in their basic methods of analysis.

This distinction between "functional" and "historical" rests on Dobzhansky's articulation of the epistemological connection between microevolution and macroevolution—namely that we can study functional evolutionary mechanisms scientifically (including experimentally) only over the short term, using living organisms; fields such as systematics and (especially) paleontology examine only historical patterns, past results of actual evolutionary history. Even if we view history as a grand "natural experiment" that has already been run, we understand history to be a connected sequence of unique events. It becomes the task of historical science to elucidate that history, while it is the task of functional science to understand the mechanisms underlying such histories.

However, much misunderstanding arises if we see science divided into two supposedly different camps, the one examining function, the other history. For example, students of phylogenetic history (systematists and paleontologists) sometimes complain about the *generality* of natural selection. Natural selection is understood to produce both stability and modification in the phenotypic properties of organisms; it seems useless as an explanatory device when it comes to understanding why the one particular course of historical stability and change—of all that might have been—in fact occurred. Put another way, *any* historical pattern would be explained in precisely the same way, as the outcome of an interplay of random and deterministic processes affecting gene content and frequency within organisms and populations through time.

Systematists and paleontologists have too readily accepted the distinction between historical and functional science. Indeed, there are even reasons to believe that there is no such useful distinction to be drawn at all. For one thing, as ensuing chapters of this book will stress, there are recurring *patterns* of stability and change through time, patterns that embrace genetic change, as well as organismic phenotypic change, and the composition of species within monophyletic taxa. Such patterns are *classes of recurrent phenomena;* as such, in contrast with isolated events, they are much more readily linked to processes—evolutionary dynamics—that are fairly well understood. As an example, parallel and convergent evolution (similar adaptations appearing in distantly related organisms living in similar ecological situations) produce patterns of similarity which lend themselves to explanation in functional, adaptive terms.

Yet there is an even deeper reason to view the supposed distinction between historical and functional science with suspicion. The task of any science, as physicist Max Planck pointed out many years ago, is simply to describe the material universe; both to describe its physical components and to elucidate the processes of interaction among its components. All material entities have two basic properties: spatio-temporal distribution and the potential, at least, for some form of interaction with other such entities. "Spatiotemporal distribution" simply means that entities are bounded in time as well as in space. Subatomic particles have ephemeral (by human standards) histories; they have evanescent manifestations inside cloud chambers, before they join together within the nucleus of an atom. And we are misled, as well, by the usual activities of physicists and chemists studying properties of atoms and molecules. When characterizing the physicochemical properties of water, the fact that each water molecule has had a history is generally irrelevant, yet it is true. It is also conceivable that the history of formation of particular water molecules could be of interest, and even approachable given the right conditions. But, in general, a chemist wants to discover those properties of water that hold true of any water molecule, under certain standard conditions. It is this functional approach which yields the sorts of generalities we call scientific *laws*.

If all entities have histories, and if functionalists simply ignore unique histories to elucidate general properties of classes of entities (such as "all water molecules at standard temperature and pressure"), we nonetheless have not yet liberated "historical" scientists from their (largely self-imposed) roles as documentors of unique historical events. To demonstrate that there is indeed no truly meaningful distinction between functional and historical science, we need to show that there are entities of truly large scale—distributed widely in space and particularly through time—entities moreover that also have the potential of interaction. Should such biological entities exist, then the possibility exists for the "historical" branch of biology to contribute in a "functional" manner to describing entities that exist in general in biological nature, and to understanding the processes underlying their interactions and producing their histories.

As an example (and as I shall discuss in detail in Chap. 4), species have been variously regarded simply as collections of similar organisms, or as integrated, functional entities in which component organisms are bound together through a network of reproductive activity. The latter view sees species as a category of biological entity, each example of which is spatiotemporally bounded. In particular, every species is seen to have a birth and a death. If species are not construed as entities—as Mayr (1942) has remarked—then there is little reason to discuss the process of their birth. *Speciation theory,* as Ghiselin (1987, p. 129) points out, is a perfect example of a theory of a general, functional process that arises as a subject of legitimate theoretical concern if and only if we see the category "species" as composed of a number (at least 10 million in the living biota) of different particular entities that nonetheless all share attributes in common. As we shall see in Chap. 4, Darwin did not see species as entities and hence omitted discussion of the "origin of species" in his book of that very title.

Thus the resolution to the apparent contrast—and conflict— between so-called historical and functional science is simply to see that in the material universe (biotic as well as abiotic), entities exist that vary in their spatiotemporal dimensions. The case for seeing various entities such as species, monophyletic taxa, and ecological communities and ecosystems as real entities is discussed in later chapters. For the moment, suffice it to say that, because of their longer characteristic time constants, species and monophyletic taxa cannot be studied in conventional experimental ways; processes characteristic of such large-scale entities can be approached only by adopting the epistemological stance that sees recurrent patterns within categories of such extant and extinct large-scale biological entities.

Genic and Organismic Macroevolution

Even this brief examination of epistemological and ontological issues in evolution is enough to show that our simple definition of macroevolution developed in the opening pages of this chapter needs to be refined. After all, "large-scale" genetic change can potentially, at least, be developed very quickly. And molecular biologists, probing the inner structure and workings of the genome, have recently added to the catalogue of processes biasing the retention and transmission of genetic information—processes intrinsic to the genome itself, and not mediated by the external environment (as is the case in natural selection). Such intrinsic processes constitute a separate, genic level in the evolutionary process. In contrast, the focus of this book is on the original (and still very much central) question of evolutionary biology: the explanation of phenotypic diversity and the design apparent in nature (the adaptive "fit" of organisms to their environments) approached through analysis of the biotic and physical environmental context of such change. Genic phenomena—such as Dover's (1982) "molecular drive," in which processes intrinsic to the genome bias the replication and transmission of genetic information—are clearly important to evolution but lie largely beyond the scope of this book. Ontogenetic phenomena, as when small-scale mutational change early in ontogeny is said to have "cascading" macroevolutionary effects as ontogeny proceeds, likewise will not be discussed in any detail herein. Genic and ontogenetic aspects of macroevolutionary theory are discussed more fully in Levinton (1988).

"Organismic macroevolution," of course, is closely tied to "genic macroevolution," as both seek to explain large-scale modifications of the phenotypes of organisms. But the term "organismic macroevolution" refers mostly to the accumulation of phenotypic (and underlying genotypic) change in organisms that results from their living in aggregates, groups variously called *populations* or *demes*. The term refers, as well, to the one-to-one match between an organism and its surrounding biotic and abiotic environment, which include, of course, the conspecifics of a local population, plus all other organisms of the local ecosystem, and the physicochemical parameters of the abiotic world. That match between organism and environment—as incomplete and imperfect as it may often seem—prompted Darwin's formulation of a theory of adaptive change through natural selection. In modern terms, selection works on existing, genetically based phenotypic variation. Such variation is maintained by a number of genetic processes (e.g., recombination) acting within organisms and arises ultimately from mutation; thus organismic evolution is intimately linked to within-organismic processes. The random process of genetic drift also enters in as a refinement of understanding genetic processes at the population level. Selection and, to a lesser extent, genetic drift are the key processes of modern evolutionary biology, held to produce small-scale change over the short run and long-term macroevolutionary change over the long run of geological time. It is this level that has historically formed the core of (macro)evolutionary theory, and the one that we shall examine in some detail in Chaps. 2 and 3.

Taxic Macroevolution

No one in modern biology disputes the basic knowledge concerning the material existence of DNA, RNA, triplet base pairs, codons, chromosomes, and, of course, organisms, though much remains to be learned about the structure and functioning of the genome. Thus we see the intrinsic evolutionary importance of studying the natures of these categories of entities and the interactive processes in which they are involved.

With "taxic" macroevolution, however, there is room for legitimate disagreement. On the one hand, macroevolution has been treated in the evolutionary synthesis as virtually synonymous with evolution of taxa of higher categorical rank (or the "higher categories," as they were erroneously called until Simpson, 1963, drew attention to the important distinction between "taxon" and "category"). Yet, as is clear from study of the details of the works of Dobzhansky, Mayr, Simpson, and the German biologist Bernhard Rensch, their theories were not so much about taxa as about the origin of the organismic phenotypic features by which we define and recognize such taxa. Rensch's book *Neuere Probleme der Abstammungslehre* (1947), translated into English in 1960 as *Evolution Above the Species Level,* was written during World War II without knowledge of the earlier writings of the evolutionary synthesis; it is concerned almost wholly with the nature of adaptive transformation of organismic phenotypic features. Throughout, Rensch repeatedly asks—and answers affirmatively—whether the small-scale processes of evolutionary change are sufficient to account for the large-scale changes observed in evolutionary history.

On the other hand, much of the recent literature (particularly within paleontology, or "paleobiology,") concerns taxa per se—be it patterns of diversity change within *clades* (i.e., large-scale taxa, whether or not explicitly monophyletic) or putative mechanisms of such taxic diversity change, as in the discussions of "species selection," "species sorting," or the "effect hypothesis" (see Chap. 5 and Vrba and Eldredge, 1984, for a review). Most such discussions implicitly (or even explicitly) view species and taxa of higher categorical rank as real entities. But it is important to realize that there are sound epistemological reasons for taking such efforts seriously even if the basic ontological assertion that taxa (including species) are real genealogical entities, in effect large-scale entities of genetic information, is not accepted. For as the work of the early contributors to the evolutionary synthesis makes clear (and, indeed, as Darwin's original discussion also makes abundantly obvious), taxic names provide handy means of referring to adaptations that have been inherited by large numbers of descendants.

Thus, whether by "mammal" one has in mind the organismic traits that define Mammalia—hair, mammary glands, etc.—or the entire skein of (known and unknown) species that have descended from the first species with those traits will prove to make a big difference in the particular theory of macroevolution one will prefer. Yet, on epistemological grounds alone, all evolutionary biologists will concede that taxa such as Mammalia have something to do with the concept of macroevolution.

Traditional organismic macroevolutionary theory perceives taxa as collections of organisms (and species) sharing unity of descent, but focuses on the history of the adaptive characteristics (the defining features) of those taxa. From this viewpoint, "taxic macroevolution" has little or no ontological significance. In contrast, "taxic macroevolution" as used in this book sees (monophyletic) taxa literally as branches (of various lengths and thicknesses) of the phylogenetic tree

of life. Such "higher" taxa are strings of two or more genealogically connected species. Such a formulation invites theoretical analysis and empirical investigation of a variety of phenomena, such as replacement of a major taxon by another following an episode of mass extinction, as when Mammalia, extant for at least 135 million years while archosaurian "reptiles" dominated terrestrial habitats, themselves underwent a succession of radiations in the Tertiary, following the extinctions at the Cretaceous-Tertiary boundary. Such phenomena have long been familiar to evolutionary biologists. But there is little, to date, in the way of general theories or "laws" (comparable, e.g., to "allopatric speciation" or "recombination") that embrace extinction of a taxon and subsequent radiation of another. Such theories can only arise if evolutionary biologists look for recurrent patterns, and if large-scale biological entities such as species and monophyletic taxa are taken seriously as real entities in nature.

But there is an even more direct, and profound, connection between organismic and taxic macroevolution. As discussed extensively in Chaps. 4 and 5, species are in many ways a unique kind of taxon. The nature and structural organization as well as the mode of origination of species are intricately related to the more general problem of adaptive stasis and change of organismic phenotypic characteristics. Such taxic considerations provide much of the context for understanding why, when, and how much adaptive change occurs in evolutionary history.

In recent years, macroevolutionary theorists have begun to focus on biological hierarchies. The genealogical and ecological hierarchies are of special significance to an analysis of the evolutionary process. In the genealogical hierarchy, organisms, through their reproductive activities, are parts of species; species, in turn, are parts of higher taxa— monophyletic lineages of two or more species. By the same token, the economic activities of organisms (i.e., those actions related to energy capture, conversion, and utilization) lead them to be associated into local populations; such local populations have ecological niches, as they interact with the physical environment and with other, non-conspecific local populations, forming local ecosystems. Local ecosystems, in turn, are associated with other such systems to form larger-scale, regional ecosystems. Much of contemporary macroevolutionary theory is geared to understanding the nature of the entities within these hierarchies, and interactions within and between these levels within each hierarchy, and, especially, *between* hierarchies.

The distinction between economic and genealogical processes—seen clearly at the organism as well as at higher levels—is crucial to any modern discussion of macroevolution. Earlier studies tended not to make such a distinction explicit; however, it begins to appear in this book in Chaps. 2 and 3. In Chaps. 4 and 5 (on the nature of species, the connection between reproductive adaptive change [speciation] and economic adaptive change, and models of species selection and sorting), the distinction between economic and genealogical phenotypic properties assumes a critical role in the analysis.

Finally, in Chaps. 6 and 7, respectively, I address larger-scale genealogical and ecological macroevolutionary patterns, including aspects of hierarchy theory. Chapter 8 offers a summary of the main points and arguments of the book.

The Integration of Macroevolutionary Theory

We return to epistemology as a final word of introduction to macroevolution. Biologists differ in their fields of expertise, and in the corresponding interests that they bring to the subject of evolution. Molecular geneticists are necessarily entranced with the fine intricacies of construction and function of the complex molecules of heredity; population geneticists are equally drawn to the complexities of the fates of genes within populations, and they also see the beautiful simplicity of many recurrent patterns that help make nature seem intelligible. Functional morphologists and ethologists come the closest of modern biologists to devoting their research to Darwin's original problem: design in nature, known in evolutionary circles simply as *adaptation*. Systematists and paleontologists focus their attention on species and larger-scale taxa, for which they have a keen regard; and ecologists, with their interest in the dynamic integration of biological entities on a moment-by-moment basis, see the adaptations of organisms, but also larger-scale economic units—communities and ecosystems—that also have a direct (if as yet under-explored) bearing on the evolutionary process, including macroevolution.

The point of all this, of course, is that all these areas of biological investigation are relevant to an understanding of evolution. We cannot divide the pie and claim that "microevolution" is solely the province of geneticists, while systematists and paleontologists study "macroevolution." Neither can we claim that somehow it is all one and only the geneticist can deal directly with both entities and processes that figure into the puzzle of evolutionary mechanisms. The trick, as I see it, is to recognize a series of levels of biological entities, each with its own intrinsic processes, and effects that it exerts on higher and lower entities. But this is a matter of ontology, and still somewhat controversial. The practical, epistemological side that benefits us all is that we can look at the input of these several disciplines, characterize the basic position that each takes on macroevolution, and summarize the progress and contribution that each makes to the total picture of macroevolution on its own merits. For there is no one theory of macroevolution, and each discipline has a part to contribute to a complete understanding of what macroevolution is all about.

Notes to Chapter 1

1. It is important to recognize that when biologists write that "populations evolve," they are actually referring to the traits of organisms within those populations. When organismic traits are modified in kind and frequency through time, a population is said to have evolved. However, it is the traits and their underlying genetic information which have changed, i.e., "evolved."

2. Also known as the *modern synthesis* or the *synthetic theory of evolution*, the evolutionary synthesis is taken here as the basis of modern evolutionary theory. For an important collection of essays bearing on the history and nature of the synthesis, see Mayr and Provine (1980); for a critical analysis of four important early books that led to the synthesis (i.e., Dobzhansky, 1937a, 1941; Mayr, 1942; Simpson 1944), see Eldredge (1985a).

3. *Epistemology* is that branch of philosophy that deals with the nature of knowledge claims; in science, epistemology is a virtual synonym of methodological theory, e.g., experimental protocol in genetics, or cladistics (phylogenetic systematics) in the analysis of phylogenetic history. In contrast, *ontology* concerns the actual nature of entities that exist in the real world. Science seeks to describe such entities. The importance of these two related but distinctly different branches of philosophy to evolution will be stressed throughout the remainder of this book.

Chapter 2

Adaptation and Organismic Macroevolution I: The Modern Synthesis and the Transformation of Morphology

Dobzhansky's formulation in 1937—that we must place "a sign of equality" between microevolution and macroevolution—set the stage for a conceptual unification, or synthesis, between the recently forged understanding of the genetic basis of adaptive evolution and the large-scale, long-term changes in the evolutionary history of life. There were several direct, epistemological consequences of adopting Dobzhansky's view. The first, already mentioned in Chap. 1, was the advantage that such a position offered for placing the study of adaptation through natural selection squarely within the realm of empirical science. Natural selection works on a generation-by-generation basis; members of the species *Homo sapiens,* with their lifetimes of 3 score and 10 years (longer than the generation spans of most other organisms), can devise experimental protocols, or set up observational opportunities in the wild, that will yield data on the intensity and effects of natural selection (Endler, 1986).

A more subtle but no less direct consequence of adoption of Dobzhansky's approach, however, was the comparative neglect of macroevolutionary theory after an initial burst of work as the modern synthesis was being forged. In particular, until recently there has been little formal analysis of what the nature of adaptive transformation of organismic phenotypic properties might be. There are two general approaches to such a problem: (1) theoretical analysis of patterns or rates of adaptive change that would accrue through geological time as the result of general considerations of the adaptive model, and (2) analysis of actual patterns of phenotypic stability and modification in geological time. The two approaches are, of course, by no means mutually exclusive, and in most analyses, elements of both are evident.

It has been known since Darwin's day that rates of phenotypic transformation vary both within and between lineages through time. Elephants have undergone more change than opossums in the last 50 million years. Lungfish underwent rapid diversification soon after they arose in the Middle Devonian; rates of lungfish morphological evolution fell drastically thereafter, and lungfish today are considered classic examples of "living fossils," having undergone very little change in the past 350 million years (Westoll, 1949). And as brain size was rapidly increasing within our own hominid lineage, the number of fingers and toes remained constant, at the primitive complement established in the Carboniferous in the early days of tetrapod vertebrate history.

It is the task of macroevolutionary theory focused on the adaptive transformation of phenotypic features to consider precisely how generation-by-generation selection works over the long term to fashion large-scale modifications in adaptations. Such considerations very naturally would include statements of tempo—rates of change, including the conditions and factors under which rates would be expected to vary. However, the most essential feature of the adaptive model of macroevolutionary transformation is implicit in Dobzhansky's statement itself: an understanding of how selection works to modify gene frequencies within a population on a generation-to-generation basis is simply extrapolated over many generations to yield a picture of long-term transformation of correspondingly greater order of magnitude than the amount of change observable experimentally or in the wild in natural populations in ecological time.

Again, it was Theodosius Dobzhansky, writing in the third edition of his *Genetics and the Origin of Species* (1951), who outlined the model in its simplest, clearest, and perhaps most elegant terms. Dobzhansky equated the present-day diversity of life with ecological niches; the origin of the diversity springs from the modification of niches, and in particular the fragmentation of niches through time. Central to his model of the adaptive history of life is Wright's (1932) notion of the *adaptive landscape,* by all odds the most important metaphor in macroevolutionary theory of the past 50 years. Dobzhansky's model is as follows (Dobzhansky, 1951, pp. 9–10):

The enormous diversity of organisms may be envisaged as correlated with the immense variety of environments and of ecological niches which exist on earth. But the variety of ecological niches is not only immense, it is also discontinuous. One species of insect may feed on, for example, oak leaves, and another species on pine needles; an insect intermediate between oak and pine would probably starve to death. Hence, the living world is not a formless array of randomly combining genes and traits, but a great array of families of related gene combinations, which are clustered on a large but finite number of adaptive peaks. Each living species may be thought of as occupying one of the available peaks in the field of gene combinations. The adaptive valleys are deserted and empty.

Furthermore, the adaptive peaks and valleys are not interspersed at random. "Adjacent" adaptive peaks are arranged in groups, which may be likened to mountain ranges in which the separate pinnacles are divided by relatively shallow notches. Thus, the ecological niche occupied by the species "lion" is relatively much closer to those occupied by tiger, puma, and leopard than to those occupied by wolf, coyote, and jackal. The feline adaptive peaks form a group different from the group of canine "peaks." But the feline, canine, ursine, musteline, and certain other groups of peaks form together the adaptive "range" of carnivores, which is separated by deep adaptive valleys from the "ranges" of rodents, bats, ungulates, primates, and others. In turn, these ranges are again members of the adaptive system of mammals, which are ecologically and biologically segregated, as a group, from the adaptive systems of birds, reptiles, etc. The hierarchic nature of the biological classification reflects the objectively ascertainable discontinuity of adaptive niches, in other words the discontinuity of ways and means by which organisms that inhabit the world derive their livelihood from the environment.

Macroevolution—from the perspective of the adaptive transformation of organismic phenotypes—has been seen overwhelmingly as a matter of tracking adaptive peaks (which are sometimes seen as equivalents of ecological niches) as those peaks change position through geological time. It is to the adaptive landscape, with its peaks and valleys, that we now turn.

The Adaptive Landscape

It was Sewall Wright, in 1932, who first formulated the notion of the adaptive landscape. Wright was concerned to illustrate the multivariate situation in which thousands of loci, each with several alleles, would, upon recombination, yield a diverse array of organisms in each generation. Some of these allelic combinations were bound to be more "harmonious" than others, as Wright put it (Wright, 1932, p. 358). Though the circumstances he described were multidimensional, Wright hit upon the idea of depicting such combinations on a direct analogue of a two-dimensional topographical map, on which the "more harmonious" allelic combinations were represented as hills, or peaks, and the less favorable combinations as valleys. Each population within each species would have many peaks and valleys. The problem of evolution, as Wright said he saw it in 1932, was for a species to maximize the number of combinations on the relatively higher peaks in the available field of allelic combinations.

Wright's formulation became part of his *shifting balance theory;* Wright (best known as a mathematically gifted geneticist devoted to the analysis of breeding data and the problems of purely mathematical population genetics) saw species in nature for the most part as divided into what he first called *colonies* (later referring to them as *demes*). His description of nature—at least insofar as sexually reproducing organisms are concerned—has been controversial, though probably more accurate than most writers (with the important exception of Dobzhansky) have been willing to grant. The shifting balance theory addresses the different histories undergone within each deme, the history of a species representing the totality of those within-deme histories. Demes could be variously expected to become modified adaptively, to merge with other demes, or to become extinct. In any case, at least in 1932, Wright saw the process of maximizing the number of harmonious allelic combinations on the relatively higher peaks in the field to be less a matter of natural selection than the result of chance, one version of his formulation of "genetic drift."

We will encounter Wright's shifting balance theory as we consider within-species evolutionary events in greater detail in Chap. 3. The point to be developed at the moment is that beginning to some degree with Wright himself (e.g., Wright, 1932), but especially with Dobzhansky (especially 1937a, 1941, and 1951; see also Mayr, 1942, and Simpson, 1944), a tendency quickly developed to modify Wright's original use of the adaptive landscape metaphor. Rather than seeing a peak for each harmonious gene combination, there was instead a movement to depict populations and even *entire species* on a single peak, as is graphically illustrated in Dobzhansky's verbal imagery in the passage quoted in the previous section. In macroevolutionary theory, peaks in the adaptive landscape became firmly equated with the niches of entire species. Within microevolutionary theory—specifically, within population genetics—an allied use of Wright's original formulation of the adaptive landscape (the *fitness landscape*) remains in use. Occasionally, as in Stenseth and Maynard Smith's (1984) use of the fitness landscape in their discussion of Van Valen's (1973) Red Queen hypothesis, the two uses of landscape surfaces in evolutionary imagery and analysis converge, as we shall see in Chap. 3.

The gist of the modern conceptualization of macroevolution stems from Dobzhansky, who wrote (1937a, p. 186) that he could "hardly eschew" sketching the outlines of a general theory of evolution. Starting with his expansion of Wright's metaphor of adaptive peaks and valleys, Dobzhansky visualized "each living species or race...as occupying one of the available peaks in the field of gene combinations" (Dobzhansky, 1937a, p. 187). Such a species, faced with environmental change, would either become extinct or be forced to undergo a reconstruction of its collective genotype, fashioning gene combinations suitable to the modified environmental conditions. Alternatively, a species might "find its way from one of the adaptive peaks to the others in the available field."

Thus there are two basic models of adaptive change: either natural selection (and, especially in evolutionary theories of the 1930s, the less directed, hit-or-miss processes of genetic drift) will track environmental change, modifying the phenotypic properties of organisms as an adaptive response to that environmental change, or a species (or a portion of a species) may change position in the adaptive landscape, whether in response to environmental change or not. The latter model was particularly attractive to macroevolutionary theorists, as it afforded a means of handling the apparent suddenness of the appearance of taxa of relatively high rank in the fossil record. The process of switching between two adaptive peaks forms the very heart of George Gaylord Simpson's theory of *quantum evolution*.

Simpson's Theory of Quantum Evolution

The role of macroevolutionary theorist in the early days of the evolutionary synthesis fell to paleontologist G. G. Simpson. Both Dobzhansky and Mayr, in their early books, which were among the core documents of the synthesis (Dobzhansky, 1937a, 1941, and Mayr, 1942—see Eldredge, 1985a, for extensive discussions of these books), included discussions of macroevolutionary phenomena and outlines of a theory of macroevolutionary processes. Indeed, Dobzhansky (1941, p. 343) included a brief presentation which anticipated Simpson's discussion of quantum evolution in several important ways. Nonetheless, because it is paleontologists who deal directly with the results of the evolutionary process in geological time (however imperfectly these events may be represented in the rock record), it was to paleontologist Simpson that the opportunity fell for constructing a theory that harmonized the emerging principles of neo-Darwinian adaptive evolution with patterns of events in the history of life. Simpson seized the opportunity, insisting in his *Tempo and Mode in Evolution* that the very nature of the historical events in geological time necessitated a theory that integrated what he called the "evolutionary determinants" in ways not anticipated by geneticists, who deal with small-scale, short-term evolutionary phenomena. To Simpson in 1944, it was by no means a straightforward task simply to extrapolate the known mechanisms of adaptive microevolution to explain the evolutionary history of life in adaptive terms. The patterns of life's history demand a somewhat novel concatenation of genetic parameters and processes to yield an accurate macroevolutionary theory. Though the theory he devised in 1944 was, at least in some respects, an extreme version of present-day macroevolutionary theory, the details of Simpson's early theory are nonetheless important as the earliest extensive discussion of macroevolution in explicitly neo-Darwinian terms, and, as such, a forerunner of contemporary macroevolutionary theory.

Perhaps Simpson's most important contribution to evolutionary theory was his recognition that there are gaps in the fossil record, gaps that in many cases may reflect the very nature of evolutionary processes at least as much as deficiencies in the formation, preservation, recovery and study of fossils. Darwin's (1859, Chap. 9) discussion of the imperfections of the geological record laid the groundwork for the field of *taphonomy,* which is concerned with how the fossil record is actually formed. It was known since the nineteenth century that only a fraction of geological time is ever recorded in actual sedimentary rock strata: if a body of rock represents the passage of a million years from the time its oldest sedimentary grains were deposited up through the moment when the last grains were laid down, the intervening strata, no matter how thick, record as a rule far less than half the elapsed time. There are simply longer intervals of time when no sediments are accumulated than there are moments when deposition occurs. This salient fact—plus all the vagaries that enter into a living organism's dying in the right place, becoming buried prior to decay and mechanical and chemical decomposition, further resisting destruction as a fossil, and ultimately becoming exposed, collected, and studied—conspires automatically to render the fossil record full of gaps.

Simpson suggested—as had Dobzhansky (1941) briefly before him; indeed, the theme goes back to Darwin—that the gaps perceived between low-level taxonomic groups such as species and genera almost always reflect the artifact of such geologically induced gaps. But, he went on, gaps between families and taxa of even higher rank could not be so easily explained as the mere artifacts of a poor fossil record. Most families, orders, classes, and phyla appear rather suddenly in the fossil record, often without anatomically intermediate forms smoothly interlinking evolutionarily derived descendant taxa with their presumed ancestors. Whales and bats, for example, appear in the Eocene; while the earliest known members of each order are somewhat primitive vis-à-vis later whales and bats, respectively, nonetheless those first known fossils are recognizably members of those orders: they are most definitely not intermediate forms between some group of ancestral mammals and the whales or bats.

But the crucial point to Simpson's argument was this: Whereas the gaps between species and genera involve sufficiently minor amounts of anatomical change so that typical patterns of rather abrupt appearance of descendants necessitates no modification of standard neo-Darwinian theory, the gaps between higher taxa are another matter. If, Simpson argued, we invoke gradual adaptive modification at rates customarily observed between species and genera to explain the evolutionary origins of whales and bats, we would require scores, and in some cases even hundreds, of millions of years. Clearly this is impossible: both bats and whales were derived from ground-dwelling placental mammals, two ancestral taxa that could not themselves have arisen much before the end of the Cretaceous, or even the Paleocene—perhaps as few as a scant 10 million years before the earliest known bats and whales had lived. It seemed obvious to Simpson that some special combination of evolutionary factors is implicated in the origin of taxa of higher categorical rank. And that special set of factors combine to produce evolutionary change at very high rates indeed. Theory led Simpson to conclude that the gaps between higher taxa must reflect unusually high rates of evolutionary change.

Simpson's list of evolutionary determinants—the factors that account for evolutionary change—contained no surprises: "variability, rate and character of mutations, length of generations, size of populations, and natural selection." It is in his characterization of natural selection that the reader first encounters the adaptive landscape in Simpson's book. He writes (1944, pp. 89–90), "The model of centripetal selection is a symmetrical, pointed peak and of centrifugal selection, a complementary negative feature, a basin. Positions on uniform slopes or dip-surfaces have purely linear selection. The whole landscape is a complex of the three elements, none in entirely pure form." Simpson depicted the landscape in constant motion, "at times more like a choppy sea than a static landscape"; but, after all, the motion is generally slow, and so could be compared, after all, "with a landscape that is being eroded, rejuvenated, and so forth, rather than with a fluid surface" (Simpson, 1944, p. 90; see fig. 2.1).

Simpson developed a model, *quantum evolution,* to characterize the causal pathways that enable a population or species (Simpson did not discriminate between the two very closely) to change from one adaptive peak to another. His term "quantum" was borrowed from its use in physics, where atoms abruptly jump from one energy level to the next, reflecting the orbital position of electrons. Simpson felt that, in

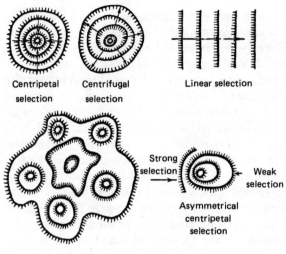

Centripetal   Centrifugal   Linear selection
selection   selection

Strong
selection →   Weak
                     selection

Asymmetrical
centripetal
selection

Fractionating selection

Figure 2.1 Simpson's depiction of "selection landscapes. Contours are analgous to those of topographical maps, with hachures placed on the downhill side. The direction of selection is uphill, and intensity is proportional to slope." (Redrawn from Simpson, 1944, Fig. 11, p. 90)

view of the very high rates of anatomical transformation implied by the paleontological gaps between closely related taxa of high categorical rank, small populations must be involved in the transition between two adaptive peaks. Small populations would simultaneously account for two factors: (1) the lack of commonly preserved (anatomical) intermediates between ancestral and descendant taxa and (2) the rapid rate of evolution.

In his earliest statement of quantum evolution, Simpson also argued that small population size would facilitate *genetic drift*. Simpson (and Dobzhansky as well, but for different reasons) was drawn to the idea of genetic drift to explain the *loss* of adaptation that the metaphor of *leaving* an adaptive peak seemed to call for.

In 1944, Simpson's theory of quantum evolution was divided into three sequential steps. In phase 1, there is a loss of adaptation, an *inadaptive* phase, brought about by random factors, specifically genetic drift, followed by phase 2, a *preadaptive* phase, in which the population, now between adaptive peaks, survives long enough to find itself with the sufficient requisite (and favorable) variation so that in phase 3, selection takes over and rapidly shapes the population for occupation of the new, adjacent adaptive peak.

Later, apparently largely in response to criticisms leveled by Wright (1945) in a book review of Simpson (1944) against Simpson's use of genetic models (particularly genetic drift) and by Schaeffer (1948) on aspects of artiodactyl evolution, Simpson (1953) abandoned his "formerly more extreme views," seeing quantum evolution simply as a subset of phyletic evolution, albeit involving moderate- to small-size populations undergoing rapid evolutionary change. As Gould (e.g., 1980b) has convincingly argued, it was only as the evolutionary synthesis "hardened" and its most prominent contributors drew conceptually closer in the late 1940s and early 1950s that the greater variety of evolutionary factors was diminished, and natural selection began to stand virtually alone as a causal evolutionary mechanism. In reducing his threefold scheme of inadaptive, preadaptive, and adaptive phases of quantum evolution to a single phase of rapid, linear modification under strong natural selection, Simpson was bringing his model of large-scale evolutionary modifications of adaptation more in line with the selectionist views of Dobzhansky, Mayr, and other evolutionary theorists of the day.

Quantum evolution, in Simpson's theory of 1944, was but one of three evolutionary modes, the other two being *speciation* (or, simply, *splitting* in his later writing) and *phyletic evolution*, i.e., transformation of genetic and phenotypic properties of organisms within a lineage through time without any splitting of the lineage. The three modes corresponded, to some extent, to two additional tripartite classifications in Simpson's *Tempo and Mode in Evolution*. In one, Simpson distinguished microevolution, macroevolution, and megaevolution—where microevolution involves population-level, generation-by-generation processes, macroevolution involves processes leading to the appearance of new species and genera, and megaevolution pertains to the appearance of families and taxa of even higher categorical rank.

In yet another tripartite scheme, Simpson argued that there are three independent distributions of evolutionary rates (i.e., rates of transformation of phenotypic organismic properties): a normally distributed set of average rates (*horotely*), as well as a distinct set of abnormally slow and unusually rapid rates (*bradytely* and *tachytely*, respectively). Because unusually rapid rates of evolution are marked characteristically by an *absence* of data (rapidly evolving populations tend to leave a scant fossil record, or none at all), Simpson claimed that study of bradytely, the inverse situation of large populations evolving unusually slowly, will shed light on the characteristics and underlying causal factors of tachytely. Thus tachytely is intimately associated with Simpson's original model of quantum evolution—and quantum evolution is usually, if not solely, implicated in the origin of taxa of relatively high categorical rank—the phenomenon he elsewhere in the 1944 book dubbed "megaevolution."

Simpson (1944) utilized the features of equid (horse) phylogeny to illustrate (in his Chap. 2) his use of the adaptive landscape and, later (in his Chaps. 6 and 7), his concept of the adaptive zone and quantum evolution. As will become evident in a later chapter in this book (Chap. 6), interpretations of phylogeny, which serve, in a sense, as the data used to test hypotheses of evolutionary mechanisms, are themselves complex hypotheses. The accuracy of such phylogenetic reconstructions determines to a very great extent the accuracy and utility of the evolutionary theory put forth as a causal explanation of that phylogeny. Phylogenies simply must be accurate representations of patterns of large-scale evolutionary events. It further matters very much what methodology is followed in elucidating a phylogenetic hypothesis. Simpson's equid phylogeny as presented in his discussions of 1944 represents what has been termed a *scenario*—complex statements of genealogical descent, ancestral and descendant relationships among taxa (in this case, of higher categorical rank), and adaptive characteristics of component organisms, and taxa, involved. In Chap. 6, when the topic of phylogenetic pattern is addressed more fully, a distinction will be drawn between a hypothesis of genealogy (as simply depicted on cladograms[1]), the more complex notion of *phylogenetic trees* (where some taxa are held to be ancestral to others), and scenarios such as Simpson was concerned to draw for horse evolution. As will become apparent in that discussion, the only Linnaean category (rank) containing taxa that are ancestors and descendants in the evolutionary process is that of the species. Though such considerations render Simpson's discussions of equid phylogeny and underlying evolutionary causation difficult to interpret, his discussions are worth following as they illustrate the general pattern of macroevolutionary theorizing, centered in the general notion of adaptation, that has until recently dominated evolutionary theory in this sphere.

Simpson on Horse Evolution

Figure 2.2 is based on Simpson's illustration of equid phylogeny imposed on a two-peaked adaptive landscape in each of four successive time slices. The peaks represent major feeding types: browsing and grazing. Judging from their dentitions, the earliest horses were all browsers; all modern horses are grazers. Thus, at some point during equid phylogeny, grazing was developed. Also at some point browsing disappeared. That the two points were not one and the same, i.e., that browsers did not become "extinct by transformation" into grazers, is shown by the coexistence of browsing and grazing horses during much of the Miocene epoch. Obviously, *some* horses adopted a grazing habit,

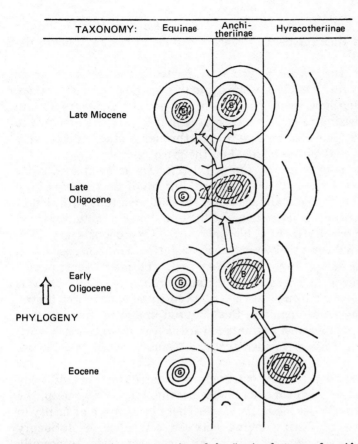

| TAXONOMY: | Equinae | Anchi-theriinae | Hyracotheriinae |

Figure 2.2 Simpson's representation of the "major features of equid phylogeny" as "the movement of populations on a dynamic selection landscape." Compare with Fig. 2.4. (Redrawn from Simpson, 1944, Fig. 13, p. 92)

a shift from the ancestral feeding habit that is well correlated with the spread of siliceous grasses as an available food source in the mid-Tertiary.

Simpson (1944, pp. 91ff.; 1953, pp. 158ff.) couched his essentially neo-Darwinian explanation of how such an adaptive shift could occur in the temporal specifics of horse evolution. Note that in equating an equid feeding type with an adaptive peak, Simpson saw peaks more as large-scale analogues of ecological niches than as harmonious genetic combinations manifested in the phenotypes of individual organisms. As figure 2.2 shows, it is higher-level taxa (subfamilies, two of them nonmonophyletic; see MacFadden, 1976) that occupy the peaks. Taxa, from species up through the Linnaean hierarchy, are thus visualized as occupying large-scale versions of ecological niches—further implying that taxa themselves play concerted roles in the economy of nature.

To Simpson, the grazing peak clearly existed in the Eocene, but was unoccupied by any members of the equid lineage. The "problem," then, was to imagine how some members of the equid clade were able to leave the browsing peak, to which horses in general were assumed to be well adapted, and to manage to pass through a stage of relatively ill adaptation and gain a foothold on the grazing peak.

Simpson's scenario on how the peak shift was accomplished is instructive—and, though the details are difficult if not impossible to verify, probably in the main accurate. He imagined that variation in browsing dentitions in Eocene and Oligocene horses was to some extent asymmetrical. Grazing horses evolved hypsodont (very high crowned) teeth during their subsequent evolution. Simpson speculated that selection among early browsers was in the main "centripetal," what is now generally termed *stabilizing selection*. Variants towards higher- and lower-crowned teeth (i.e., than those optimal for browsing) would be selected against. But Simpson imagined that selection would be stronger against variants towards *lower*-crowned teeth; variations towards higher-crowned teeth, of course, would take horses closer to the grazing peak.

Higher-crowned teeth are positively correlated with overall body size in horses: through time, as horses became larger in general, the relative length of their teeth increased. There is always a difficulty in such instances of distinguishing between coincident evolutionary change and the correlations induced by a common factor, especially simple growth and body size. For it may well be that higher-crowned teeth are simply an accidental by-product of prolonged growth to relatively larger body sizes, quite apart from the fact that high-crowned teeth last longer during the lifetime of a horse subjected to the high rate of molar wear induced by siliceous grasses. Indeed, it is this pattern of correlated growth that Simpson invoked to explain variation further towards the grazing peak in Oligocene horses: as body size increased, variation towards higher-crowned molars followed suit as "secondary adaptations" to higher body size, and thus variation was "incidentally" in the direction of the grazing peak.

Thus, because of asymmetrical selection and variation towards higher-crowned teeth as a simple correlate of increased body size, Simpson saw the two peaks coming closer to one another so that, by the late Oligocene or early Miocene, they were close enough that some variant horse individuals found themselves in the valley between the two peaks. Note that the grazing peak is depicted as stationary; it is the browsing peak which is seen to have changed position. Presumably, however, this change actually lies in the modal adaptations of browsing horses, in particular (presumably) their modal body size and concomitant variation (especially in molar crown height). There is no suggestion in Simpson's discussion that nonhorse biotic or abiotic components of the adaptive peak were themselves changing.

Once the variant horses were roughly equidistant from the tops of the two feeding peaks, they found themselves subject to "centrifugal" selection in two directions, i.e., some towards the grazing peak, the others back towards the browsing peak. The animals themselves, in other words, were in Simpson's view relatively "ill-adapted." Simpson (1944, p. 53) felt that those "that gained the slope leading to grazing were, with relative suddenness, subjected to strong selection away from browsing. This slope is steeper than those of the browsing peak, and the grazing peak is higher"—assertions difficult to evaluate, certainly, but based on Simpson's conclusion that grazing represents a specialization (behaviorally and anatomically) that would be difficult to reverse or further modify. Selection drove this "population" further up the grazing slope, so that by the end of the Miocene, the peak had been attained. Thereafter, the two types of horse remained quite distinct (each with its minor variations); browsers themselves failed to adjust to changing conditions and became extinct by the end of the Tertiary, an event that was wholly divorced from the events and underlying causal processes that saw grazers evolve from browsers much earlier on.

Simpson's example is well chosen: a sort of "mid-range" example of adaptive change, involving a clear-cut ecological distinction that is reflected in equally pronounced behavioral and anatomical modifications in the evolutionary history of a group. Involving more than the relatively slight changes that generally accompany speciation, yet not as dramatically large-scale as, for example, the origin of flight in archosaurs or mammals, the example is apt because the functional anatomical significance of the different morphologies is fairly clear as was the phylogeny itself—at least in terms of the general level at which Simpson discusses it.

Though subfamilially ranked taxa are depicted as the occupants of the two adaptive peaks, and terms such as "population" appear in the discussion, it is also evident that the focus of the discussion—the actual goal—is the explanation of the transformation of anatomical form in a specifically adaptive context. This is especially clear in Simpson's equation of a shift in position of the browsing peak with anatomical modification within the browsing lineage. Uniquely held anatomical properties define taxa in systematics; the origin, maintenance, and modification of those characteristics are the focus of evolutionary theory, and any discussion of the origin, evolutionary histories, and eventual extinctions of taxa are in fact discussions about the organismic properties that are used to define and recognize those taxa. To Simpson, at least in the context of evolutionary theory, taxic names are purely expedients to refer to phylogenetically connected collections of organisms that share homologous traits that are similar to differing degrees.

Simpson was not alone in the synthesis in treating macroevolution strictly as a problem in the transformation of anatomical characteristics of organisms. Yet he did not go along with what (as we shall later see) was probably the greatest departure from traditional Darwinism that was to emerge with the modern synthesis: the notion that species are real entities, reproductive communities each with their own origins, histories, and terminations. Thus, that higher taxa are utilized only as "modal" summaries of the adaptations of organisms (in the case of equid evolution, of their basic feeding types) in Simpson's treatment agrees well with the earlier-cited imagery that Dobzhansky provided in 1951—in which the entire history of life is explained with reference to a single grand adaptive landscape. But in not incorporating species (for one reason because he felt that speciation represents lower-level, and generally trivial, amounts of adaptive phenotypic change), Simpson was able to frame his discussion of macroevolution strictly in terms of variation and selection, ignoring the discontinuity in adaptive differentiation that both Dobzhansky (1937a, 1941) and Mayr (1942) saw that speciation injects into the evolutionary process.

Later in *Tempo and Mode in Evolution,* Simpson returned to horse evolution, this time as an explicit illustration of his theory of quantum evolution. As can be seen in Fig. 2.3, Simpson characterized his three main modes of evolution in terms of the *adaptive grid,* on which one or more *adaptive zones* could be depicted. Speciation, to Simpson, involves the exploitation of *subzones* within a general adaptive zone, while phyletic evolution involves some concerted change in adaptations, though the lineage remains within the confines of a zone, which itself is seen to undergo some degree of change. Quantum evolution represents the shift from one adaptive zone to another and is in many respects the same metaphor as Simpson's concept of the shift between adaptive peaks, as his discussion of equid phylogeny in terms of adaptive zones and quantum evolution makes abundantly clear.

Figure 2.4 is based on Simpson's depiction of equid evolution in terms of adaptive zones and quantum evolution. Note that in contrast to his earlier diagram showing a shift in the actual position of the browsing peak, in his later discussion, the positions of the grazing and browsing zones remain constant, while it is the adaptive complex represented by a population of horses that does the actual shifting. The shift, as already mentioned, involves an *inadaptive phase* (in which

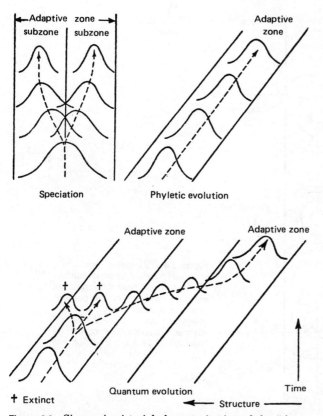

Figure 2.3 Simpson's pictorial characterization of the "three major modes of evolution...Broken lines represent phylogeny, and the frequency curves represent the populations in successive stages." (Redrawn from Simpson, 1944, Fig. 31, p. 198)

the browsing adaptation is lost) and a *preadaptive phase* (essentially corresponding to the period Simpson imagined, in which a population relatively ill-adapted in the valley between the two peaks finds itself able to graze by virtue of its incidentally acquired variation in the direction of hypsodonty). Once the horses begin grazing, they enter the *adaptive phase,* as selection rapidly moves them up the steep slope towards the grazing peak. Thus the three phases of quantum evolution fit in nicely with Simpson's earlier discussion of coincidental variation in the shift from one adaptive peak to another. However, there is more of an explicit statement of "all-or-none" change in quantum evolution than appears in his earlier discussions of shift between adaptive peaks.

Simpson (1953), as already mentioned, later dropped the inadaptive and preadaptive phases to quantum evolution. In line with the emerg-

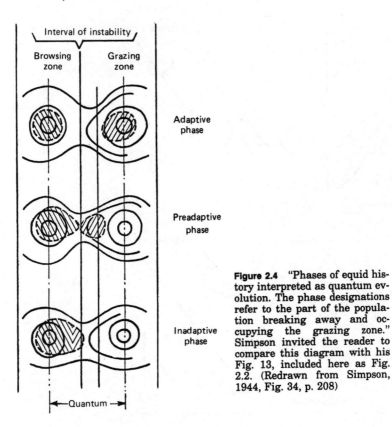

Figure 2.4 "Phases of equid history interpreted as quantum evolution. The phase designations refer to the part of the population breaking away and occupying the grazing zone." Simpson invited the reader to compare this diagram with his Fig. 13, included here as Fig. 2.2. (Redrawn from Simpson, 1944, Fig. 34, p. 208)

ing orthodoxy of strict selectionism, Simpson's later version of quantum evolution amounted to an "extreme, more-or-less limiting case of phyletic evolution." In this later version of quantum evolution, selection simply acts with great intensity and rapidity to effect large-scale adaptive change. In his earlier discussions, the basic shift in adaptation in horse evolution was accomplished relatively rapidly, while much longer periods of time were required for elaborating that change—for climbing the peak towards adaptive perfection. In the later model, splitting of lineages is not particularly required, as it is in the earlier models; gone, too, is the requirement that the essential change is rapid vis-à-vis a longer period of less rapid change. Simpson's earlier statements were much more specific than those made later about the timing and context of events of major adaptive change in evolution. The details of Simpson's particular model of how that change occurs are open to criticism; but lack of attention to the details of timing and circumstance characteristic of actual events of adaptive change has caused evolutionary theory over the past 40 years to remain vaguer than it could have been on the nature of macroevolutionary adaptive change.

Macroevolutionary Transformation: Trends

Directionality is inherent in any consideration of evolutionary history and the processes underlying that history. It could hardly be otherwise: we are interested in explaining how some phenotypic state arose from some other state, as the original and still the most commonly asked kind of question in evolutionary biology. How did birds come to be equipped with feathers and the ability to fly? How did the complex social systems of some hymenopteran insects evolve? How did the placenta of eutherian mammals develop? In each of these examples, the structure, function, or behavior to be explained clearly arose from some more primitive state (by definition). Such a state, moreover, can be specified at least in general terms, not least because organisms of the sister clade that lack the evolutionary specializations are still extant. Examples are terrestrial diapsid reptiles (with scales instead of feathers and lacking full flight powers, though some, such as the modern lizard *Draco*, do glide); asocial hymenopterans, which, together with the vast bulk of other insects, amply demonstrate the primitive behavioral condition for insects; and egg-laying amniotes (birds and "reptiles"), which indicate that the primitive state of Amniota was probably egg laying in the external environment.

Thus, any consideration of how state *B* is derived from state *A* automatically involves a vector, a direction of change. Nor is a fossil record necessary for the idea of "trend" to enter into an analysis of evolutionary history. For example, a simple survey of extant hominid species (ourselves, *Homo sapiens;* the chimpanzees, the genus *Pan;* gorillas, *Gorilla;* orangutans, *Pongo;* and gibbons, *Hylobates*) strongly indicates that there has been an increase in both absolute and relative brain size in the lineage leading to *Homo* since that lineage diverged from that leading to whichever of the extant apes is our closest relative—tradition having it as *Pan,* but see Schwartz (1987), who makes a case for *Pongo.* We would predict, then, that cranial capacities of fossil hominids should increase through time, a prediction, moreover, that is abundantly confirmed in the fossil record of the past 4 million years (Eldredge and Tattersall, 1982). This example is discussed in greater detail when trends are considered in conjunction with species selection in Chap. 5.

As a first-order approximation, trends (whether or not they are documented in the fossil record) are explained by simple reference to the principle enunciated in 1937 by Dobzhansky (1937a): by putting a "sign of equality" between micro- and macroevolution. We know that *linear* (or *directional*) *artificial selection* can produce directional changes in various attributes of experimental organisms; we simply imagine that in the wild, linear natural selection effects long-term, larger-scale directional changes in the phenotypic properties of organisms. Long-term, directional natural selection, as we have already seen, is the basic explanatory device of evolutionary theory.

As a second-order, more-detailed consideration of how selection operates to yield directional, major change in evolution, theorists generally have resorted (as Simpson did) to the imagery of the adaptive landscape. As we have seen, there are two basic options available: either the landscape is changing, and thus the positions of peaks are modified, providing the selective impetus for adaptive change, or peaks are held to be constant in position, in which case organisms either perfect their adaptations to those peaks or change to other peaks. We will follow out some of the more recent utilizations of the adaptive landscape topography in macroevolutionary theory in greater detail in the next chapter.

For the remainder of this chapter, we will consider some of the third-order, more-detailed examinations of the transformation of phenotypic properties as provided by paleontologists, by systematists, and, particularly, by functional morphologists (anatomists). There are remarkably few such high-quality, detailed discussions in the literature of evolutionary biology. Students of behavior, including social behavior, will note the similarity in the manner and style of presentation between morphological examples and instances of transformation discussed in the several behavioral literatures. In particular, sociobiology represents a straightforward application of modern Darwinism (as discussed in detail in Chap. 3); the principles of adaptive transformation developed in more traditional areas of evolutionary concern—especially organismic morphology—are readily recognized in many sociobiological analyses.

The Transformation of Morphology

It is worth noting that although some of the earliest champions of Darwinian theory were well-known anatomists (e.g., T. H. Huxley in England and E. Haeckel in Germany), some of Darwin's most outspoken critics were equally renowned for their expertise in anatomy, systematics, and paleontology (e.g., Richard Owen of the British Museum, and L. Agassiz, who emigrated from Switzerland to found the Museum of Comparative Zoology at Harvard University in the 1840s). Reasons for either adopting or rejecting a vision of the history of life as profound and "unorthodox" as that of evolution are complex and varied from person to person. Motivations include religious beliefs, competitive jealousy, and no doubt other factors beyond simple rational contemplation of the nature of the claim and how well it fits what biologists thought they knew about the nature of living systems at the time.

Yet there is something about the study of anatomical systems per se which has often led to rather antievolutionary views: it is as if the complexity of anatomical systems poses an insurmountable obstacle to transformation. Time after time people claim not to be able to see how a certain complex structure could have arisen from a simpler state; thus it was that the vertebrate eye (or, in creationist literature, the eye of *Homo sapiens*), held to be so complex, with the precise interconnections and interfunctioning of all its parts all necessary for the organ to function properly, was held up as an almost instantaneous reaction against Darwin. The vertebrate eye remains the core example of a structure that some say is "impossible" to evolve slowly, through a series of intermediate stages, from some simpler system to its present complex state.

Yet to an evolutionist, the vertebrate eye clearly did evolve. Vertebrates are all craniates, and all those lacking eyes have close relatives *with* eyes, leading to the supposition that blindness represents secondary *loss* of eyes. But consider our closest living relatives among nonvertebrates: the chordate *Amphioxus,* which has simple light-sensitive pigmented spots—hardly an eye—in its head region. Enteropneusts (hemichordates) lack eyes; and the deuterostome echinoderms lack heads altogether. Yet vertebrates are chordates, and chordates are close relatives of echinoderms, sharing evolutionarily derived anatomical features (at the level of Deuterostomia, involving details of embryological development). And clearly, within Deuterostomia, only vertebrates have the "vertebrate" eye; indeed, (among deuterostomes) it is mostly vertebrates that have eyes at all. Clearly, the vertebrates sprang from ancestors somewhere within Deuterostomia, ancestors that lacked eyes, and perhaps even heads.

The evolutionist also realizes that the eyes of squid and octopi (cephalopod mollusks) are very similar in complexity and anatomical configuration to those of vertebrates. Yet cephalopods are mollusks. The eyes of cephalopods are not particularly similar to the eyes of snails or the light receptors of some (headless) bivalves (such as scallops); nor do they resemble the eyes of polychaete worms, which, like mollusks, belong to the Protostomia. The common ancestors of protostomes and deuterostomes (probably among the lophophorates, which include brachiopods, bryozoans, and phoronid "worms") all lack heads, let alone eyes, altogether.

Thus complex "vertebrate-type" eyes have appeared at least twice in evolutionary history. Pronouncing such transformations as a priori "impossible" is thus ruled out of court: if we accept the hypothesis that life has evolved, such structures had to be derived from simpler states. Insisting that their complexity speaks against their being evolved reflects, instead, more a poverty of imagination than any necessary conclusion drawn from a consideration of complexity of structure per se.

Thus it has fallen to evolutionary-inclined morphologists and functional anatomists to provide explanations of how transformation of anatomical features may have occurred. Though there has been a strong tendency in recent years to belittle such attempts to frame coherent explanations of anatomical transformation (they are often derided as "Just So Stories"), the tradition of this explanation arises largely as a reaction against the antievolution position that such transformation *cannot* have occurred in the first place.

Morphologists have two basic options in approaching an analysis of evolutionary transformations. They may frame their study strictly to encompass known morphological states, where a series of anatomical (structural *and* functional) states are held to be transitional between a primitive and an ultimately derived condition. These states may be found in a series of fossils, or in a mixture of fossil and Recent taxa, or may be known (at least in detail) only through a series of living taxa (as in one of the examples given below). Alternatively, in the absence of any known intermediate stages, morphologists tackling a particular problem of evolutionary transformation may resort to an analysis of a carefully constructed series of *hypothetical* intermediate stages, an admittedly riskier proposition, as *saltational* models use the absence of known intermediate stages as direct indication that none ever existed. Saltational models of morphological transformation share the feature that large-scale changes occur as single-step events; the models differ among themselves on how large the steps are, how rapidly they occur, and how they are in fact effected. An example of a largely hypothetical situation consistent with mainstream evolutionary theory—Bock's (1965, 1979) analysis of the origin of birds and, specifically, bird flight—is presented below. Naturally, many studies combine both approaches: for example, the evolution of the vertebrate eye is usually discussed by showing how intermediate stages of complexity leading to the fully fledged vertebrate eye are both imaginable and supported by some comparative anatomical and embryological evidence.

Moreover, anatomists have tended to remain conservative; the complexity of a structure is often seen as a constraining, limiting force of the possibilities of change. Not only must new structure be fashioned from what already exists, but the modification of developmental pathways to lead to such new structures is itself seen as difficult to accomplish. Developmental pathways are complex and delicate; too much disruption yields inviable offspring rather than usefully new adult structures.

At its best, then, functional anatomical analyses that form the basis of transformational scenarios are derived with a full appreciation of (1) the complexity of the structures, (2) their current mode of function, and (3) the limitations on modification placed on an anatomical system by past conditions of that system. With this in mind, we can review some examples of macroevolutionary analysis as presented by some functional morphologists who are also systematists and paleontologists.

The Origin of Bird Flight

Bock (1965, 1979) has analyzed the evolutionary development of avian flight in an explicit context of macroevolutionary theory. Bock, an avian comparative and functional anatomist, has written that evolutionary theory in general is weak on the details of how macroevolutionary transformation can be understood as a sequential series of microevolutionary steps reducible to the principles of the neo-Darwinian paradigm of natural selection working on within-population, genetically based variation (Bock, 1979, p. 20). Though in some contributions (e.g., 1970, 1972, with a summary in 1979) Bock has stressed the importance of speciation in macroevolution, it is actually the diversity of species, leading to interspecific interactions of various sorts which acts as sources of (natural) "selection forces" that he considers important, rather than speciation per se, as developed in later chapters of this book. Macroevolution, whether it be the transformation of single features or the origin of entire taxa, is "simply the consequence of additive microevolutionary change" according to Bock (1979, p. 67).

One approach Bock (e.g., 1979) has advocated for testing concepts of evolutionary adaptation is the notion of "pseudophylogenies," in which series of closely related species (e.g., of Hawaiian honeycreepers, family Drepanididae) display a spectrum of states of transformation of one or more morphological features. Such a series mimics the phyletic series that underlies patterns of macroevolutionary change; at the very least, the persistence of such a suite of features in closely allied species demonstrates the plausibility of interpreting the transformation as a continuum of intergradational morphological intermediates, rather than a result of a single morphological "leap," as postulated in various saltational models. The existence of such a sequence also aids the morphologist considerably in the task of positing likely intermediate stages in the transformational sequence.

Bock (1979) has criticized Simpson's (original 1944) model of quantum evolution because, in common with saltational models, it involves no intermediate *stable* taxa with organisms successfully adapted to a niche somewhere between the starting and end points of the transformational series under analysis. To Bock (1979), all steps in such a macroevolutionary sequence are adaptive and under the control of directional natural selection; his model obviously contrasts with Simpson's initial formulation of an inadaptive (and preadaptive, a concept Bock endorses) phase.

Thus, to Bock, macroevolutionary transformation works because it produces a series of functional intermediate stages which are adaptations in their own right. His analysis of the origin of flight in birds is a case in point. Bock (1965, 1979) imagines a series of successive transitions from "bipedal locomotion" to an "arboreal" mode, then on to a "leaping," followed by a "gliding" mode of life, which is the final stage achieved before full flight. While the transition from quadrupedal locomotion to full-fledged flight is great, the transitions between stable states in Bock's outline of bird evolution represent considerably more modest changes, readily imagined as the outcome of episodes of directional natural selection.

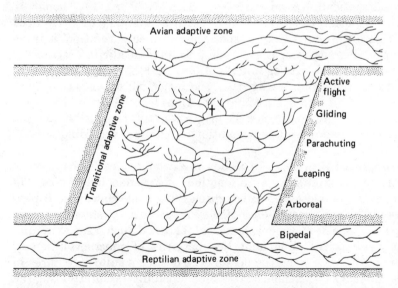

Figure 2.5   Bock's "composite model for the adaptive origin of a new group of organisms, in this case the evolution of birds from reptiles. The successive radiations seen in the transitional adaptive zone form a pattern of stepwise evolutionary levels indicated on the side of the transitional zone. The approximate position of *Archaeopteryx* is indicated by a cross (†). Relative widths of the major and transitional zones, sites of the various radiations, and relative times are not shown to correct proportions."

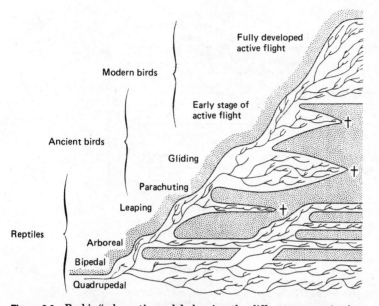

Modern birds

Fully developed
active flight

Early stage of
active flight

Ancient birds

Gliding

Parachuting

Leaping

Reptiles

Arboreal

Bipedal

Quadrupedal

Figure 2.6 Bock's "schematic model showing the different stages in the evolution of birds through successive taxonomic groups—reptiles, ancient birds, and modern birds. The possibilities of transitional zones appearing several times and of their continued existence, for example, at the arboreal and leaping levels, are emphasized in this model. Moreover, the model illustrates the severe selection pressure exerted by flying birds on other arboreal groups that may be evolving fully developed aerial adaptations." (Redrawn from Bock, 1979, Fig. 16, p. 54)

Bock illustrated his model in a series of figures, two of which are reproduced here (Figs. 2.5 and 2.6). One of them (Fig. 2.5), illustrating schematically the branching sequence of speciations underlying the phylogeny, depicts the macroevolutionary transition as extending from the "reptilian adaptive zone" to the "avian adaptive zone," but extending through the several stages as different lineages speciate and exploit the various levels of the "transitional adaptive zone." Thus Bock has adopted Simpson's notion of an adaptive zone and used it in his own analysis.

In Fig. 2.6, we see Bock's (1979, Fig. 16) addition of taxon names (albeit informally) to the transformational scheme. Here, however, there is depicted a persistent lineage leading from "quadrupedal" to "fully developed active flight." The intermediate levels are depicted here as stable zones, each of which lead, in due course, to extinction (except later arboreal invasions by reptiles). This figure agrees closely with Simpson's (1944, 1953) discussion of *"Ahnenreihen"* and *"Stufenreihen,"* i.e., the explanation of "pseudo-orthogenetic lines" as

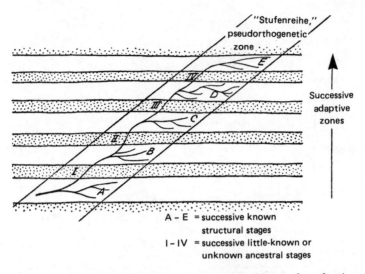

Figure 2.7 Simpson's "diagrammatic representation on the adaptive grid of the steplike evolution of a group through successive occupation of different adaptive zones. The series *A–E* are *Stufenreihen* and may be taken as an orthogenetic series, although in fact the direction of evolution in each stage is not towards the next stage. This is, however, a reflection and to some extent an approximation of the undiscovered truly ancestral sequence, I–IV, the evolution of which is approximately rectilinear." (Redrawn from Simpson, 1944, Fig. 29, p. 194)

really a series of stable invasions of "successive adaptive zones" (Fig. 2.7). Consideration of the nature of species and the role of speciation in governing adaptive transformation (see Chaps. 4 and 5) yields a picture reminiscent in some ways of Simpson's discussion of "*Stufenreihen*" and Bock's concept of multiple levels.

Transformation of Feeding Mechanisms in Catfish

Bock's phylogeny of the Drepanididae was "pseudo" only in the sense that it did not involve a direct sequence of ancestors and descendants. Most observers do agree that Drepanididae are a natural, or *monophyletic,* taxon. Moreover, it is in principle true that there is a pattern of relationships within the extant members of Drepanididae such that any given species shares a more recent common ancestry with one other particular species than with any other. In other words, there is a network of *recency of common ancestry* interlinking all living species of Drepanididae. Particularly because, in the speciation process, ancestral species generally live on alongside descendants, the derivation of a scheme of relationships among species within a monophyletic group in fact amounts to positing a true phylogeny. The investigator must always bear in mind, however, that through extinction, intermediate species may indeed be missing from the array under study.

Evolutionary morphologist George Lauder begins his analyses of evolutionary transformations with a *cladogram* detailing the relationships among the taxa under analysis. In their study of the historical transformation of functional design of the feeding mechanisms of loricarioid catfish, Schaefer and Lauder (1986) mapped the distribution of "structural novelties" onto a cladogram of relationships among the five families of Loricarioidea that they recognize. The cladogram (Fig. 2.8) was derived independently (i.e., by other workers) using characters other than those of the structural–functional complex of the feeding mechanism. Schaefer and Lauder (1986) identify three levels of increasing complexity in the evolution of loricarioid feeding mechanisms, and these correlate to a high degree with the nodes joining families (or, in one case, with the origin of the most derived family Loricariidae) on the cladogram. Thus "plateaus of stability" exist, defined by the retention of a level of structural and functional morphology by a number of species within a large-scale monophyletic taxon.

In their analysis, Schaefer and Lauder (1986) recognize a primitive loricarioid condition, characteristic of Nematogenyidae and Trichomycteridae; the first stage of advance, characteristic of Callichthyidae, Astroblepidae, and Loricariidae, is retained in its simplest (primitive) form only in Callichthyidae. The next level is represented by Astroblepidae and Loricariidae, while the latter family defines a final, (so far) most advanced level of structural–functional design of the feeding mechanism. Thus the levels of structural–functional transformation agree very well with the cladogram, which is of the simple "pectinate" form, with progressively more plesiomorphic (primitive) taxa rooted to the cladogram to the left of coordinate, derived sister taxa.

The use of families (rather than species) would appear coarse-grained with respect to the problem of relating the reconstructed historical sequence to processes underlying the adaptive transformation of structures and associated functions. That each of the structural–functional novelties appeared in the stem species common to all subsequent descendants in the various monophyletic subtaxa of the Loricarioidea is assumed. The advantage of this approach, of course, is that actual structural–functional stages of a transformation series are addressed in the analysis, without recourse to reconstruction of hypothetical intermediate levels, as is necessary, e.g., in Bock's (1965, 1979) consideration of the origin of flight in birds. The main problem in the Schaefer and Lauder (1986) study is to analyze the actual di-

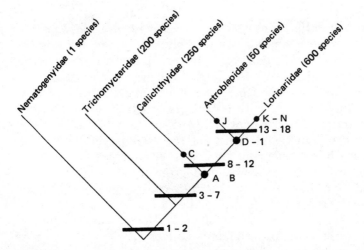

Figure 2.8 Schaefer and Lauder's cladogram (redrawn) depicting phylogenetic relationships among families of loricarioid catfish. Numbered characters are those derived from other sources to support the cladogram; lettered characters are those mapped onto the cladogram derived from original study by Schaefer and Lauder. (From Schaefer and Lauder, 1986, Fig. 2, p. 492; characters detailed in Appendix II, pp. 507–508)

rection, nature, and pattern of the structural–functional transformation(s) themselves. Schaefer and Lauder were able to elucidate a general trend from their analysis of stages of the transformation of loricarioid feeding mechanisms, and it is in the demonstration of such trends that a more concrete connection between theory and analysis of a real-world sequence of (macro)evolutionary transformation is most easily seen.

In brief, Schaefer and Lauder postulate three basic stages of evolutionary transformation beyond the primitive condition. In the first (in the lineage leading to Callichthyidae, Astroblepidae, and Loricariidae), a highly mobile premaxilla was acquired. Next (Astroblepidae and Loricariidae) new muscle insertions were added to the highly mobile premaxilla, and movements were attained that were independent of maxillary movements. There were also coordinate changes that increased mobility of the lower jaw. Finally, in the lineage leading to the family Loricariidae, a portion of the jaw adductor muscle became inserted on the premaxilla.

Schaefer and Lauder conclude that there was an increase in the number of "biomechanical pathways" in both upper and lower jaws of loricarioids. Structural–functional trends include a "decoupling of primitively constrained systems" (i.e., a freeing of the premaxilla and symphysis of the lower jaw), increase in the number of "biomechanical linkage systems" (i.e., with new muscle insertions on the premaxilla), and "an increased multiplicity of biomechanical pathways controlling functional components in the feeding mechanism."

The authors associate such freeing up of previously constrained systems (with subsequent additional interconnections) with morphological and trophic (i.e., modes of feeding) diversity. Specifically, they claim (Schaefer and Lauder, 1986, p. 489) that a "decoupling of previously constrained systems leads to increased morphological and structural (anatomical) diversity in descendant species."

Thus, in confronting a system recording the transformation of a structural–functional complex, in which intermediate stages are represented at least in part by organisms still extant, the emphasis of the investigators, at least in this case, focuses on (1) the rearrangement of structural parts per se and (2) the constraints that ancestral configurations impose on further modifications of the system. Absence of more detailed and explicitly historical sequences prompts such a prudent focus and introduces some further evolutionary considerations arising out of comparative and functional anatomy: so-called key innovations and the more general notion of *"Bauplan."*

Key Innovations, Bauplans, and Adaptive Radiations

In postulating that characteristic patterns of structural and functional change (specifically, freeing of previously constrained items of morphology) allow a complexification of biomechanical pathways, Schaefer and Lauder (1986) are building on an old theme in evolutionary morphology: the double-sided issue of *constraints* and *triggers* of adaptive change that arise from morphological configurations themselves. What is at issue is causal control of stability and change of anatomical systems. To some degree, such control arises from genetic and morphogenetic levels. But in the transformation of adult morphology, ancestral anatomical configurations determine in large measure what can and cannot—thus to some extent what will and will not—happen in the way of transformation into descendant morphologies.

When such causal control is seen as a limiting, conservative factor, the term "constraint" is appropriate. But the opposite theme—in which the causal control is seen as an allowance of possibilities for further and, occasionally, significant change—is that the ancestral morphology is seen to act more like a *trigger* to further change. Such was the significance attached by Schaefer and Lauder to changes in the feeding mechanisms of loricarioid catfishes: a freeing of biomechanical elements was interpreted to have induced (or at least made possible) a radiation into a variety of new trophic modes, reflected in a heightened diversity of anatomical structures.

Simpson (1959a) termed anatomical novelties that seem to set off a great deal of further evolution *key innovations.* Citing the work of Schaeffer (1948), for example, Simpson argued that the artiodactyl (even-toed ungulate) astragalus (ankle bone), constructed in such a way as to act like a pulley, absorbing all the weight along the median axis of each foot, set the stage for the explosion of artiodactyl taxa. Artiodactyls are still the dominant mammalian herbivores; they include the extant deer, bovids (which include antelope in addition to cattle, goats, and sheep), pigs, and camels, plus a number of extinct taxa. According to Schaeffer (1948) and Simpson (1959a, p. 265), it was the appearance of the artiodactyl astragalus, allowing high-speed running essential for flight from carnivores, that signalled the success of the artiodactyls and allowed them to radiate into a variety of different ecological situations.

Many taxa seem to be composed of species that appear, at least as anatomists tend to look at them, as if they are all variations on a common theme. Pre-Darwinian anatomists were accustomed to deriving the "archetype" for a group—a sort of anatomical least common denominator from which all observed anatomical variants can be imagined to have been derived.[2] After 1859, as seen especially in the work of the German zoologist Ernst Haeckel, the concept of "common ancestor" was simply substituted for the older, preevolutionary idea of archetype. Another term that stands as a virtual synonym is the German *Bauplan,* referring to the basic structural plan common to all taxa within a monophyletic taxon; a bauplan serves as a sort of template to the anatomical diversity subsequently evolved within the group.

Bauplans (or *Baupläne* in German) serve a specific role in evolutionary morphology. For just like "key innovations," it is the development of a critical stage of anatomical design—a bauplan—in phylogeny that is said to trigger an entire "adaptive radiation," which we can define at this juncture simply as a proliferation of anatomical diversity, particularly when more than a single direction of transformation is involved, as in a "trend." For example, the derivation of the ecologically and anatomically diverse array of terrestrial marsupial mammals in Australia is a classic example of an adaptive radiation; other, more precise connotations of the term will emerge in a subsequent discussion of adaptive radiations in Chap. 6.

Whether or not "archetypal plans" or "bauplans" in fact act as catalysts for subsequent evolutionary radiation and innovation depends to some extent on how we envision the acquisition of anatomical change in phylogeny. All echinoderms, for example, share a mesodermally derived skeletal system composed of porous single-crystal plates of magnesium-rich calcium carbonate. (Some holothurians have secondarily lost an encasing hard skeleton, but nevertheless retain ossicles of this nature.) All living echinoderms, and all extinct taxa save a very few among the earliest, are characterized by a pentarradial plan of symmetry. We may specify these, and other attributes, common to all echinoderms as their sine qua non, constituting their fundamental bauplan. These features, acquired in the basic early radiation of deuterostome metazoan phylogeny, "allowed" echinoderms to exploit a variety of potential niches in the world's marine habitats for the past 575 million years.

Alternatively, we may simply see the acquisition of these basic echinoderm features as occurring very early on in the phylogenetic history of this lineage, thus supplying the structural novelties (*synapomorphies* in the context of cladistics—see Chap. 6) that serve to unite all echinoderms into a single genealogical lineage: a monophyletic taxon. From the viewpoint of evolutionary mechanisms, such novelties become primitively retained similarities (*symplesiomorphies*) throughout the rest of echinoderm history—and may as well be imagined as constraints limiting anatomical modification as much as the key features that prompted subsequent anatomical modifications.

In any case, many phylogenies are reminiscent of the picture of feeding mechanics evolution of the jaws of loricarioid catfish as presented by Schaefer and Lauder (1986) and outlined above: evolutionary novelties are not added all at once, typically, nor do subdivisions of monophyletic taxa (such as the various classes and subphyla of echinoderms) all spring *separately* from a single, ancestral source. Rather, novelties seem to accrue one by one, seriatim, often but by no means exclusively in a "pectinate" fashion, resulting in a nested pattern of relatedness among subtaxa within a monophyletic clade. Nonetheless, there are instances in which at least the living subtaxa within a well-defined monophyletic taxon do appear to represent largely separate "directions" of anatomical transformation from a common ancestor. Whether or not the ancestral morphology is taken as a constraint on, or a trigger for, further diversification is extremely difficult to decide with echinoderms, or, for that matter, with any monophyletic taxon known. We shall now examine in some detail one such putative case, that of the protostome phylum Mollusca.

A bauplan example: urmollusk and the origin of molluscan classes

Mollusks, as Morton (1958) has pointed out, have long elicited description of an archetype, an "arch-mollusk" that combines the features seen in the disparate living classes: Scaphopoda ("tusk shells"), Bivalvia (clams), Gastropoda (snails), Cephalopoda (octopi, squid, and pearly nautilus), Amphineura (chitons), and the recently discovered Monoplacophora (so far lacking a colloquial name). Molluscan phylogeny was in all likelihood even richer than its present-day diversity would indicate, as at least some of the extinct classes described by paleontologists over the years are probably correctly attributed to the phylum. Nonetheless, we will confine our attention to the morphological diversity of the six extant classes, as it is they that present by far the richest details of molluscan anatomical organization.

This discussion of the *Urmollusk* follows Morton (1958), simply because his is an especially clear presentation, and not because his version is necessarily more complete, accurate, or otherwise superior to the many other versions available. (Actually, Morton wrote his book just before the full details of the anatomy of the then–recently dredged *Neopilina galatheae*—the first described species of living monoplacophoran—had become available; such information has a deep bearing on any reconstruction of the arch-mollusk, particularly over the issue of metameric segmentation.) As in most such treatments, the *Urmollusk* is a handy heuristic device, serving as an introduction to many of the major anatomical features that characterize one or another of the major subgroups (in this case, molluscan classes) to be treated in ensuing discussions. Yet it is also clear that the archetype represents at least an approximation of both (1) an organism that can be imagined to have functioned, i.e., actually to have lived, and (2) a bauplan from which all variant versions of molluscan anatomy can be readily derived. Such a reconstruction would, of course, also minimize the number of parallel evolutionary modifications (transformations as well as outright losses of anatomical features), in keeping with the principle of parsimony in the analysis of transformation series in phylogenetic analysis (see Chap. 6).

Morton (1958; see fig. 2.9) saw the arch-mollusk possessing a simple cap-shaped shell of calcium carbonate; he saw it as a slow-moving animal probably clinging to a hard substrate with its large foot mass. Ecologically and at least superficially anatomically, such a primitive mollusk most closely resembles modern prosobranch gastropod limpets, as well as modern and (especially) Paleozoic Monoplacophora. The animal had a head (forming, with the foot, a cephalopedal mass much like that of gastropods, chitons, and monoplacophorans). Morton

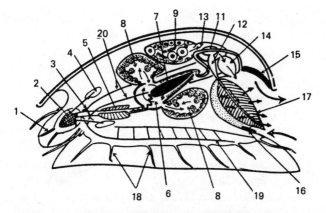

Figure 2.9 Morton's conception of the "ideal early mollusk, in side view. (1) jaws in buccal cavity, (2) radula on odontophore, (3) nerve ring, (4) salivary glands, (5) esophageal glands, (6) stomach, (7) protostyle with food string, (8) paired digestive diverticula, (9) gonad, (11) ventrical and intestine, (12) left auricle, (13) pericardium, (14) left renal organ, (15) hypobranchial gland, (16) osphradium, (17) ctenidium (showing currents), (18) epipodial tentacles, (19) pedal nerve cords, and (20) pallial nerve cords." (Redrawn from Morton, 1958, Fig., 1A, p. 13)

is silent on the possible presence of eyes: though gastropods have small eyes on tentacles on either side of the head, and cephalopods have eyes constructed along lines reminiscent of vertebrates, such organs differ materially in the details of their anatomical construction and are thus not considered *homologous* (i.e., derived from a common ancestral state). Thus there is no basis for concluding that the ancestral mollusk actually did possess eyes of any sort; presumably, if the various sorts of eyes of extant mollusks were considered homologous, Morton would have included such eyes in his reconstruction of the common ancestral mollusk. This little example of something *not* included is quite instructive, illustrating as it does the line of thought that goes into the reconstruction of a bauplan.

In general, the ancestral mollusk as depicted by Morton (1958) resembles a primitive, untorted gastropod; most extant, shelled gastropods are torted, i.e., the gut is twisted around so that the anus opensout in the same general region as the head, a necessity imposed by existence in a closed, conically tapering tube. (Shell-less gastropods are secondarily untorted.) Thus Morton shows the mantle cavity limited to the posterior region of the animal; lining the mantle cavity is the single pair of gills and the osphradium, a chemosensory organ. Most living mollusks have a single pair of gills; advanced gastropods have but a single gill. Only in the primitive cephalopod *Nautilus* are there *two* pairs of gills, taken by some early anatomists as evidence of metameric segmentation, a possible holdover from the many and repeated divisions of the annelid worm body (with which mollusks are related as protostomes). Mollusks have long been suspected of being close relatives of both annelids and arthropods, both of which are metamerically segmented; thus the presence of two pairs of gills in *Nautilus* was something of a welcome confirmation of this phylogenetic interpretation. Yet, more recent investigators tended to see those four gills as a secondarily derived duplication of an original pair, just as the eight plates of a chiton shell are obviously secondary subdivisions of an original single shell.

The discovery of *Neopilina* rather radically changed the picture of the *Urmollusk*. Many of the features traditionally predicted to be present in the arch-mollusk are in fact developed in *Neopilina;* moreover, there is unmistakable evidence for primitive metamery in monoplacophorans. There are seven or eight pairs of gills (the number varies according to species). While the status of these gills as true homologies is debated, nonetheless there are also many pairs of pedal (foot) muscle retractors; the nervous system is also segmented, with branches associated with each foot muscle mass, reinforcing a view of primary metameric segmentation. Internal organs, as well, show evidence of segmentation. Fossil evidence from the Paleozoic likewise shows the presence of multiple pairs of muscle scars, indicating that monoplacophorans were indeed primitively segmented; (monoplacophorans appear in the Cambrian, disappearing from the record at the end of the Middle Devonian period; shells of *Pilina,* very similar to those of *Neopilina* dredged from the deep sea, are known from Silurian reef environments).

It is possible to "derive" corresponding bauplans for each molluscan class from such an *Urmollusk* (perhaps a version much like Morton's, with added notions of metamery from *Neopilina*). Morton (1958) in effect does this as his discussion continues; of necessity, what emerges in such an exercise is a *mosaic* of characteristics. In bivalves and scaphopods, for example, the head is reduced; bivalves develop a hinged shell, while scaphopods elongate the shell into a tube, open at each end. Each class represents a different version of retention and modification of those features thought to be present primitively in the *Urmollusk*. Thus, of necessity, molluscan phylogeny is presented as a radiation from a single, common ancestor. Perhaps the shell, affording both protection and a substrate against which powerful muscles could work, represents the "key innovation" enabling mollusks to radiate in the variety of infaunal, epifaunal, and nektonic modes we find them in today, exploiting a wide variety of grazing, deposit feeding, filter feeding, and carnivorous habits. On the other hand, perhaps the shell and remaining features of the *Urmollusk* actually restricted molluscan evolution to rather a narrow range of possibilities—only truly exceeded as the cumbersome shell was lost (as it has been in several lineages of gastropods and in advanced cephalopods and some chitons, though shell-less "chitons" are considered separate taxa and among the most primitive mollusks in some recent phylogenetic analyses).

It is clear from this example that the connection between the elucidation of the features of a common ancestor and drawing any evolutionary implications from them is a tenuous exercise at best. Morton (1958), for one, does not attempt any such scenario building, claiming only to sketch a plausible story of pathways of anatomical transformation in early molluscan phylogeny. Indeed, characteristics of the common ancestral mollusk are likely to emerge in somewhat altered fashion from a character analysis of the sort commonly practiced in modern phylogeny reconstruction, in which patterns of relationship among subtaxa (such as the six extant molluscan classes) reveal a distribution of development of evolutionary novelty, again, rather more like that described by Schaefer and Lauder (1986). The presence of a feature in a subset of subtaxa—such as the presence of a rasping ribbon (*radula*) in the mouths of gastropods, cephalopods, and chitons—may imply retention from an *Urmollusk* (as Morton, for example, actually claims); it may also represent either (1) independent ("parallel") development (meaning that the structures are not truly homologous) or (2) development only in a lineage that led to those mollusks observed to have the structure, i.e., a feature evolved sometime later in molluscan phylogeny and shared by only some mollusks. In any case, reconstruction of ancestral anatomical configurations is clearly methodology-dependent; we will address aspects of this topic again, more fully, when the problem of modern phylogenetic analysis is discussed in Chap. 6.

Mosaic Evolution

When asked for an example of an "intermediate" form between two taxa, paleontologists traditionally point to the Upper Jurassic *Archaeopteryx,* from the Solnhofen limestone of Bavaria. De Beer (1954) studied the five known specimens and pronounced *Archaeopteryx* to be an example of what he termed "mosaic evolution." In De Beer's view, *Archaeopteryx* is an anatomical mosaic because it presents a mixture of character states that are (1) "reptilian" (e.g., it has teeth and a bony tail), (2) intermediate between reptilian and birdlike (e.g., its weakly developed sternum), and (3) fully birdlike (e.g., it possesses feathers).

All organisms are spectra of primitive and advanced (derived) characters. The large brain of *Homo sapiens* is clearly derived, while the presence of five digits on our hands and feet is a primitive feature of all tetrapods. When placed on a diagram of transition from "reptiles to birds" *Archaeopteryx* provides the useful service of providing a counterexample to the naive expectation that anatomically "intermediate" taxa must be intermediate *in all respects* between a primitive and a derived taxon. Thus De Beer's concept of mosaic evolution is a handy retort to creationists who willfully distort the point.

Yet, on a cladogram of relationships (e.g., Cracraft, 1986), *Archaeopteryx* simply falls out as the "sister group" to all other known birds, sharing the essential derived feature (synapomorphy) of feathers with all true birds, yet lacking other features of advanced birds and retaining a number of others (such as teeth) lost by most subsequent birds. In the context of such a cladogram, *Archaeopteryx* looks far less like a "missing link" between two great divisions of vertebrate life. And when seen as a particular combination of primitive and derived character states occupying a particular slot on a complex cladogram involving many different taxa, its phylogenetic neighbors appear as mosaics as well. De Beer's term is descriptively useful; it does *not,* however, describe some peculiar mode of the evolutionary process.

Adaptation: "Aptation," "Exaptation," "Preadaptation," and Related Terms and Concepts

As we have already seen, the general problem of explanation of the evolutionary origin of complex anatomical structures has long been ameliorated by the notion of *preadaptation:* structures that serve one particular function may be utilized for some unrelated function and further modified by natural selection the better to serve the second function as an adaptation. Thus Simpson invoked allometrically enlarged molars in grazing horses as a preadaptation; once the molars became sufficiently enlarged, they were suitable to be used in grazing, and selection then began rapidly to drive some horse lineages up the steep gradient of the grazing adaptive peak. Likewise, Bock foresaw climbing, parachuting, and gliding as stages in which each condition was a necessary precursor, a preadaptation that allowed the next step, culminating in full avian flight, to be developed.

Gould and Vrba (1982) have pointed to the existence of a category of anatomical and behavioral organismic properties that are "features that now enhance fitness but were not built by natural selection for their current role." The point is to make more precise the distinction between the current utility or role of a specifiable organismic pheno-

typic attribute—be it morphological, physiological, or behavioral—
and the historical development of the structure.

According to Gould and Vrba (1982), the proper term for all structures observed to increase fitness is *aptation*. An *adaptation* is an
aptation developed directly through natural selection for its current
use. On the other hand, any characteristic that developed (through
natural selection or not) that is co-opted for a new use is an *exaptation*.
Thus feathers in birds, following a suggestion of Ostrom (1979), may
have first developed as an adaptation for thermoregulation; their use
in flight may simply be a secondary effect, enabled by their presence
developed initially to serve an entirely different function. Gould and
Vrba (1982, following a suggestion from H. E. H. Paterson) also provide the example of the African black heron, which fishes by using its
wings to cast a shadow on the water, thus improving its ability to see
its prey. In such a case, the behavioral repertoire in all likelihood conforms to their restricted definition of "adaptation"; but the wings per
se were shaped by natural selection for flight.

Clearly, the notion of exaptation overlaps to some extent with previous connotations of preadaptation. Yet use of the term "preadaptation" in evolutionary biology has often suffered from an almost
mystical sense of premonitory, directional change, as if future evolutionary modifications are somehow anticipated by earlier stages of
phenotypic transformation. By choosing such clear examples—in
which utterly "co-opted" functions are so starkly different from previous functions—Gould and Vrba (1982) clarify the distinction between
current utility and mode of historical development.

Parallelism and Convergent Evolution

Biologists have long been aware that certain adaptive "designs" tend
to appear repeatedly in the course of evolutionary history. Since
Darwin, repetition in adaptive themes has stood as evidence of
thestrength of natural selection to mold similar engineering structures as a response to similar environmental conditions and concomitant organismic needs. The key feature of this pattern is that similar
phenotypes are developed more than once in evolutionary history.
When the organisms are closely related, such patterns are generally
termed *parallelisms;* when their phylogenetic histories are more remote, the pattern is called *convergence* instead. There is no hard and
fast rule of thumb that allows a clear, unambiguous distinction between parallelism and convergence, and I will treat the two terms as
virtual synonyms throughout the remainder of the discussion.

The classic example of convergent evolution is the similar, fusiform
body shape seen in many sharks, ichthyosaurs (extinct Mesozoic

aquatic "reptiles,"), and porpoises, each members of different vertebrate classes in conventional vertebrate taxonomy. From the standpoint of phylogenetic systematics (i.e., the delineation of genealogically pure lineages), recognition of a taxon consisting of sharks
+ ichthyosaurs + porpoises represents simple analytic error.
Nonetheless, from the standpoint of adaptation per se, the phenomenon of convergence (or parallelism) is important both for its general
implications on the evolutionary development of organismic design
and for its connection to some of the more extreme views taken on the
nature of adaptive aspects of the evolutionary process in recent evolutionary theory.

As we shall see in Chap. 6, refinements in the methodological theory of phylogeny reconstruction, resulting in an upsurge of phylogenetic research, confirm more than ever the rampant occurrence of
convergence (often termed *homoplasy*, or nonhomologous resemblance) in the evolutionary process. Nearly all cladograms published
in the last 15 years represent best estimates of genealogical relationships among taxa. Rarely do such patterns of relationship emerge un-
ambiguously from even the most detailed analysis: generally there is
more than one possible way to render such relationships among a series of taxa, each alternative being supported by characters held in
common by various combinations of taxa. Of the several possible
sources of analytic error (assuming, as any evolutionist must, that
there is one, and only one, correct solution to a question of phylogenetic relationships among any set of organisms), one is that the
"same" condition has evolved more than once, i.e., the systematist has
erred in assuming that the precise form of two similar structures is
homologous. For example, it would be wrong to conclude that bird,
bat, and pterosaur wings are homologous *as wings;* they *are* homologous as vertebrate forelimbs, but other characters support allocation
of birds, bats, and pterosaurs each to separate higher taxa within the
amniote tetrapod vertebrates. It is the large number of (generally less
dramatic) examples of similar situations—in which conflicts in possible attribution of relationships arise, often not at all as easily resolved
as these two vertebrate examples—that reinforces the importance of
convergence as a theme in the adaptive history of life.

Another context in which convergence becomes conspicuous lies in
an aspect (almost ironically) of *adaptive radiations:* if the primary
theme of such radiations is divergence into a number of different
modes of life from the single niche type of the common ancestor, that
radiation often produces organismic phenotypes at least superficially
similar to those encountered in other regions (or at other times in the
fossil record). Thus the classic Australian (as well as separate South
American) radiation of marsupials produced wolflike carnivores pur-

suing economic roles much like those of placental wolves of the modern biota.

Finally, and perhaps of less overall significance to major adaptive phenotypic transformation, there is the phenomenon of mimicry, in which (for several different reasons) organisms within one species come to resemble closely members of another species.

The overall theoretical importance of such patterns of parallelism and convergence is to reinforce the notion that, given the requisite variation of heritable traits, natural selection often shapes similar (even astonishingly similar) phenotypes for a variety of reasons. From this we learn that (1) there is a limited spectrum of optimal biological engineering designs for particular purposes (e.g., vertebrate flight) and (2) similar phenotypes more naturally lead to a greater incidence of close convergence (e.g., wings of various vertebrates contrasted with those of insects; but compare this with the very close resemblance between the eyes of vertebrates and those of cephalopod mollusks).

There have been, however, further theoretical analyses based on the general phenomenon of evolutionary convergence that have been argued to have a direct bearing on macroevolutionary phenomena. These discussions lie in the general area of *grades* and the polyphyletic origin of higher taxa, the concluding topic of this chapter.

Grades and Polyphyly

J. S. Huxley (1958)—who coined the term "modern synthesis," using it in a book title (Huxley, 1942)—crystallized theoretical interest in parallel evolution when he elaborated on the distinction between evolutionary *grades* and *clades*. Huxley recognized three general aspects to the evolutionary process: *cladogenesis,* or diversification (cladogenesis in most modern usages means lineage splitting); *anagenesis,* or improvement along lineages; and *stasigenesis,* or persistence. The terms refer to fates of organismic phenotypic properties: the improvement in anagenesis refers, for example, to adaptive transformation that represents some form of "evolutionary progress." Likewise, cladogenesis (i.e., in Huxley's original formulation) refers to the diversification of phenotypes, while stasigenesis refers to adaptive nonchange, or stability, similar to *stasis* (e.g., Eldredge and Gould, 1972) in discussions of the theory of punctuated equilibria (see Chaps. 3 and 4).

Huxley (1958) wished to distinguish what he saw as two separable approaches to organismic classification. Accordingly, he suggested that "clades" refer to monophyletic taxa, i.e. (especially in modern usage; see Chap. 6), all species descended from a common ancestral species. Huxley proposed the term "grades" to refer to another way of uniting clusters of species—as units of "anagenetic advance." Grades represent levels, or specifiable steps or stages, of adaptive transformation within the confines of large lineages.

Yet, as Huxley originally stressed and subsequent theorists (e.g., Simpson, 1961) elaborated, grades need not themselves be monophyletic in a strict sense. In particular, several different sublineages within the larger clade may *independently* develop in parallel the "same" (i.e., highly similar, yet not specifically homologous) phenotypic properties. We thus classify them together, even when careful analysis shows the taxon to be *polyphyletic* [which can be defined for the purposes of the present discussion simply as derivation of a higher taxon from two or more ancestral species; Simpson (1961) actually redefined "monophyly" to embrace cases of polyphyly in which all the species independently leading to the next step of a grade are members of the same higher taxon of the same or lower rank as the descendant higher taxon; see Chap. 6]. That systematists were eager to recognize that many traditionally recognized higher taxa were in fact non-monophyletic, but nonetheless valid, is a strong indication of the importance of selection-mediated adaptive change held in the minds of evolutionary biologists in the mid-1950s and 1960s. It was only shortly before this time that the modern synthesis had been completed and, in the opinions of some biologists (e.g., Gould, 1980*b;* see also Eldredge, 1985*a*), had "hardened," narrowing from a more multifarious theory to one that focused almost exclusively on adaptive transformation under the control of natural selection.

Simpson (1959*b*) reanalyzed the origin of mammals, concluding that the defining features of mammals, so far as they could be determined from fossils (especially teeth, but also cranial and postcranial skeletal anatomy, especially that of the jaw articulation and ear morphology) indicated that class Mammalia is polyphyletic. Simpson estimated that mammalian morphology arose several times in separate sublineages of the general lineage of anagenetic advance beginning with the therapsid "reptiles" of the Upper Paleozoic and Lower Mesozoic. Many subsequent authors have concluded that there is no evidence that mammalian features (e.g., the change from a quadrate-articular to a dentary-squamosal jaw articulation) evolved more than once in mammalian phylogeny. Thus all organisms, fossil and Recent, classified as "mammals" are generally now considered to belong to the same monophyletic taxon in the strictest sense of that term.

Yet there remains more to the concept of grades than a mere excessive enthusiasm for the power of natural selection leading some systematists openly to espouse the virtues of recognizing patently nonmonophyletic taxa—taxa of mixed genealogical derivation. For one thing, it was clear to Huxley (1958) and to a number of investigators who pursued his theme that many grades are in fact also clades. For example, the evolutionary history of the ammonoids (a class of externally shelled cephalopods, ranging from the Middle Devonian to the Upper Cretaceous periods) has long been read as a basic succession of three gradal groups: the Paleozoic goniatites, the Triassic ceratites, and the Jurassic-Cretaceous ammonites. The three groups differ in the complexities of their suture patterns, i.e., the lines formed by the intersection of the internal partitions and the external shell. Goniatites are the simplest, ceratites intermediate, and ammonites the most complex of all in their suture-line convolutions. Yet, as can

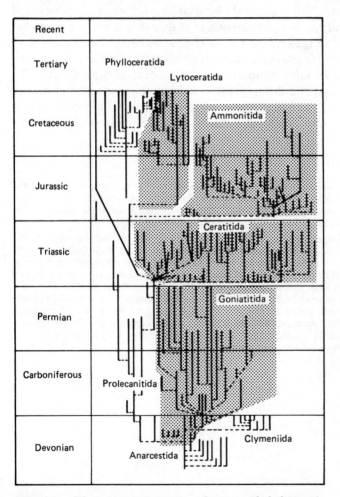

Figure 2.10 Schematic representation of ammonoid phylogenetic history. The successive goniatite, ceratite, and ammonite grades are shaded.

be seen in the diagrammatic sketch of ammonite history (Fig. 2.10), each grade is currently considered also to be (nearly) a clade; moreover, in the opinion of at least some ammonite specialists, each successive clade was derived *not* from a species within the preceding grade/clade, but from a survivor of one of the few extant lineages not included in the earlier clade which had been dominating ammonoid diversity.

Thus ammonoid history, at least, supports the notion that grades may represent separate (monophyletic) radiations within an overall lineage; just why there should be a directional transformation of the homologous character states (as in suture-line morphology) is not entirely apparent. The general similarity between grades and *Stufenreihen* and related phenomena of stages in a transformation series as reviewed in this chapter is, of course, evident. We shall return to the problem of large-scale, macroevolutionary transformation—especially *trends*—in later chapters, in the context of higher taxa. We shall see there that the differential production and survival of higher taxa (*taxic sorting*), arising from a variety of causes, becomes a factor in the explanation of large-scale directional change in evolution.

Notes to Chapter 2

1. Cladograms are diagrams depicting recency of common ancestry among a series of taxa. The methodology of phylogeny reconstruction and the contruction of cladograms is briefly discussed in Chap. 6, in conjunction with a consideration of the importance of monophyly of taxa in macroevolutionary studies.

2. It may seem incongruous that preevolutionary biology entertained the notion of "archetypes." However, the idea that anatomical diversity within monophyletic taxa reflects variations on a common theme seems to arise from the nature of the material itself, i.e., as self-evident patterns of distribution of morphology in nature. In any case, creationists have explained anatomical similarity among organisms as a manifestation of a "blueprint" used by the Creator. A hybrid version of the theme perists in contemporary creationist literature in the assertion that there is "variation within created kinds" (i.e., [micro]evolution), but not *between* "created kinds"—i.e., macroevolution does not occur according to "scientific creationism." (For more discussion of creationist tenets, see Eldredge, 1982.)

3

Adaptation and Organismic Macroevolution II: "Ultra-Darwinism" and the Rates and Timing of Adaptive Change

Historian W. B. Provine (1989) considers the evolutionary "synthesis" to be more of a "constriction" than a truly successful melding of evolutionary concepts from an assortment of biological fields, namely, genetics, systematics, paleontology, ecology, and developmental biology. Surely an important step was effected when Fisher, Haldane, and Wright showed that the findings of the first 30 years of research in genetics were in fact compatible with the older Darwinian notions of adaptive change through natural selection. Provine (1989) argues that what really happened as a consequence was a culling of much of the babble of conflicting and often contradictory causal theories that had characterized evolutionary biology for decades prior to the 1930s.

It may seem tempting to agree with Provine that little conceptually new was actually added beyond a fusion of genetics and Darwinism—a fusion that yielded the "neo-Darwinian paradigm" of natural selection acting on a groundmass of among-organism, within-population variation, the ultimate source of which is mutation. But such a historical interpretation would overlook an important point: there was at least one contribution of the early synthesis to evolutionary thought that was indeed novel, namely, the notion that species are reproductive communities and, to some extent, at least, to be construed as entities unto themselves. Crucial here were the contributions of Dobzhansky (especially 1937a) and Mayr (1942); much of the recent work in taxic macroevolution springs from their visualization of the nature of species and of the speciation process, topics we pursue in later chapters.

Notwithstanding the contributions of Dobzhansky and Mayr, and the continued interest in speciation phenomena by a number of biologists, the core of modern evolutionary theory continues to regard speciation as something of an epiphenomenon—as simply the means whereby taxic diversity is increased and phenotypic diversity perhaps maintained. Most evolutionists continue to regard the origin and further modification of adaptations as the central issue of evolutionary biology; the prevailing causal mechanism remains natural selection, working on a generation-by-generation basis within populations. Yet, for all the recent work in adaptation-centered evolutionary theory, there remains little explicit analysis of the causal pathways underlying the timing and rates of adaptive change: why—and to what extent—adaptive change occurs when it *does* occur. Though we shall review in this chapter some of the gene-centered theory that proves an exception to this generalization, the roles played by species and ecological entities such as ecosystems, acting as constraints and triggers to adaptive change, will be considered in ensuing chapters.

Indeed, far from embracing themes of species and speciation, the major shift (i.e., from basic themes of the synthesis) taken by today's "ultra-Darwinians" is to see genes as the focus of the evolutionary process. Yet many of the explanatory themes to be found in the writings of ultra-Darwinians will be familiar from earlier work reviewed in the preceding chapter. Foremost among these is the adaptive landscape, in slightly modified form, which still provides the metaphorical basis for both mathematical and qualitative analysis of evolutionary change, including the large-scale sorts of changes that fall under the rubric of "macroevolution."

Modern Darwinism

Most of modern evolutionary theory (as judged, for example, from the issues of the bimonthly journal *Evolution*) lies squarely within the realm of microevolution. The field is vibrant, as new theoretical insights (particularly, but by no means solely, in the evolution of behavior) have continued to prompt field, laboratory, and mathematical-analytic investigations. Optimality theory has been especially prevalent in the past 20 years or so; in such theory, phenotypic (in the broadest sense) features whose functions are presumed to be known are judged as ipso facto adaptations. It is commonly further assumed that selection will act to optimize such features, particularly in the face of contradictory needs of the organism. Clutch size (number of eggs laid by birds in any single reproductive episode) is a case in point. Assuming that bird couples are trying to maximize their reproductive success (and this is the central tenet of ultra-Darwinian theory), there would seem to be an optimum number of eggs to be laid per clutch. With too many eggs, viability falls off as the limits of nest size, sibling competition, and the ability of the parents to feed and otherwise care for the fledglings are exceeded. Too few eggs just as obviously reduces genic representation of the parents in the succeeding generation. Ergo, there is an ideal number of eggs—neither too few nor too many—for the average clutch for members of each species.

The value of such studies is that the details of natural selection–mediated genetic change are understood better than ever before. Selection is a generation-by-generation process, and this work utilizes precisely the sorts of data necessary to test detailed hypotheses of the action of selection in real, as well as hypothetical, situations. Nor has Dobzhansky's injunction to correlate laboratory results with carefully controlled observations in the wild been lost; Endler (1986) has recently surveyed much of the work on natural selection in the wild.

By its very nature, then, modern evolutionary biological studies focusing on adaptation and selection deal with microevolutionary adaptive change and stability. Little work is geared to bridging the conceptual gap between microevolution and macroevolution, the latter taken simply as large-scale, long-term accrual of adaptive change.

Yet some theoreticians have indeed endeavored to fill this gap. Ultra-Darwinism is a version of Darwinism that takes genes as the units of natural selection, seeing natural selection as the maximization of reproductive success as measured by the spread of genes. Beginning perhaps with biologist George Williams's (1966) *Adaptation and Natural Selection,* features of the organismic phenotype held to be adaptations are seen literally as mechanisms to favor the survival and successful reproduction of the genes underlying those characters. Williams (1966) himself was very careful to distinguish features resulting from selection as opposed to mere side effects and as such was the intellectual forerunner of Gould and Vrba's analysis of aptation, adaptation, and exaptation (see Chap. 2), as well as other suggestions reviewed later in this book.

Williams (1966) sought to place the analysis of selection and adaptation on a more rigorous and "scientific" footing. He was especially concerned to take a critical look at suggestions of *group* selection (involving analogues of natural selection acting on entire groups of organisms); his book is chiefly regarded as the Darwinian response to the idea that selection may affect entire groups as well as individual organisms within populations. As a mechanism for originating, modifying, and maintaining *organismic* adaptations, Williams's general point is certainly well taken: organismic features are shaped by organismic selection. Biotic (i.e., group-level) adaptations might justifiably be imagined to be shaped by group-level selection, but the evidence for such biotic adaptations seemed slim to Williams in 1966 and remains so to most authors to the present. We will encounter a version of this debate in Chap. 4, when we consider the notion of *species selection,* specifically promulgated in the context of recent macroevolutionary theory.

Williams (1966) also championed the notion that the gene is actually the focus of selection; at one point, he wrote (p. 68) that it is "the goal of the fox...to contribute as heavily as possible to the next generation of a fox population." Richard Dawkins's *The Selfish Gene* (1976) picked up where Williams had left off, portraying genes as almost canny entities vying for representation in the next generation, just as Darwin (1859) had seen competition for resources and mates amounting to a struggle among organisms. Yet there are important differences. To Darwin, relative reproductive success among organisms of the same sex and species within the same population was a side effect—albeit a critically important one—of the relative success each experienced as it lived its life. The "purpose" of sharp teeth in a predaceous fish, to Darwin, was to capture food items, such as other fish. Those with the strongest, sharpest teeth, all other things being equal, could be imagined to have an edge on survival, with a carryover to reproductive success, as those sharp teeth were first evolving. To a genic selectionist, however, the purpose of the sharp teeth, from an evolutionary perspective, is to confer advantage to the genes for the strongest, sharpest teeth in their race for disproportionate representation in the next generation. Such shorthand reckoning does no harm unless the unwary forgets the actual details of the causal process, as Darwin so clearly developed it.

How do ultra-Darwinians handle macroevolutionary adaptive change? Dawkins's (1986) *The Blind Watchmaker* considers the problem of adaptation in detail. Apparently writing largely in reaction to various critiques of "adaptationism" from within biology (as well as from creationists outside biology), Dawkins is at pains to reaffirm the plausibility of the Darwinian vision of incremental change accumulating under natural selection to shape the adaptations of organisms—the design in nature seen by biologist and creationist alike. Though elaborately explicit on *how* selection induces incremental change, Dawkins is almost silent on the ecological and evolutionary contexts of adaptive change, especially long-term adaptive change: the factors that promote and retard adaptive change through evolutionary time. Thus nowhere in his text, or in the writings of many contemporary evolutionary biologists, are there any theoretical models approaching the detailed complexity of those developed, e.g., by Bock (1979) and Simpson (1944, 1953), as reviewed in the previous chapter. Thus there remains a critical gap between a Darwinian-based understanding of how selection works to modify phenotypes on a generation-by-generation basis and a theory that addresses actual patterns of such change in the history of life, at least as that theory is developed by leading advocates of contemporary evolutionary theory. Actually, there *have* been attempts by some geneticists in recent years to bridge this gap, i.e., to understand through mathematical modeling just what sort of patterns of adaptive change ought to emerge over evolutionary time through selection and drift. It is to this work that we now turn.

Population Genetics and Macroevolution 1. Basic Models

While many modern evolutionists make such a stark distinction between phenotype and underlying genotype that genes per se emerge as the actual focus of selection, the mainstream of population genetics has traditionally taken a more pluralistic view. Models in population genetics are simplest if a single locus with two alleles is analyzed. More alleles and/or more loci quickly complicate the situation to the point where large computers become a necessity. Yet geneticists have long known that most phenotypic traits are polygenic: for every one trait that has a simple single-locus hereditary basis, there are hundreds more that have many loci as their genetic basis. Computational convenience rather than a simple faith that selection acts on genes per se underlies most treatments of selection on single loci in population genetics evolutionary analyses.

Geneticist Russell Lande, recognizing that the central, or at least original, problem in evolutionary theory is the explanation of change (and stability) of organismic phenotypic traits through time, has developed models explicitly geared to expressing patterns of phenotypic stasis and change. The models themselves are extensions of well-known results of population genetics, particularly the shifting balance theory of Sewall Wright, which is itself dependent upon representation of the distribution of fitness values on a mathematical surface, or *adaptive landscape* (see Chap. 2).

Wright (1931) recognized that some gene combinations are "more harmonious" than others. This is to say that some genotypes enhance survival and probability of reproductive success to a greater degree than others (at homologous loci) within populations—the concept of *relative fitness.* Relative fitness is depicted as height on a topographic map, while the planar coordinates of the map surface are alleles. (The two dimensions of the map's planar coordinate surface stand for the multidimensional array defined by all the variant allelic forms in the population.) Thus, there are typically many adaptive peaks within each population.

Wright (1931 [see also Lande, 1985, p. 7641]) showed that when fitnesses of genotypes remain constant through time (i.e., when genotypes retain the same probability for survival and reproductive success, most often imagined as a result of no environmental change), natural selection always acts to increase the *average* fitness of a population. (This result further assumes that different alleles recombine approximately independently, i.e., without the effects of linkage.) Thus a *second* adaptive landscape can be constructed, on which populations are points on a surface of *average* fitness, and where selection acts to drive populations up local adaptive peaks of mean fitness (written as $\overline{W}$, pronounced "W bar").

Wright's *shifting balance theory* considered the problem of how populations can shift from one adaptive peak to another. Populations of finite size of necessity undergo some degree of *genetic drift,* in which alleles are lost at the rate of $\frac{1}{2}N$ (where N is population size) just on chance each generation. Since selection, under the conditions given above, always acts to drive $\overline{W}$ *up* the peak, Wright considered drift, in which populations go *down* the hill and across an inadaptive valley, to be the main mechanism underlying peak shifts in evolution. As we have already seen, this is the fundamental imagery underlying Simpson's (1944) original formulation of "quantum evolution."

Lande (especially 1976, 1979, 1985, and 1986) has explicitly modified Wright's model and use of the landscape imagery to encompass polygenic phenotypic characters (rather than alleles and allelic combinations). Lande acknowledges that he is in effect supplying mathematical precision to Simpson's qualitative application of Wright's model to actual patterns of phenotypic change in evolution. As Lande wrote (1976, p. 317), "Thus Simpson's intuitive notion of adaptive zones for phenotypes was correct. His concept has been made more precise by finding that the level of adaptation is the mean fitness of individuals in the population and that the other dimensions of the adaptive zones are the average values of phenotypic characters in the population."

Lande first addressed simple patterns of linear (phyletic) transformation of quantitative phenotypic characters in examples taken from the paleontological literature. Assuming that fitness values of phenotypes remain constant (directly analogous to Wright's assumption for genotypes) and that populations are infinite, Lande adduced equations to describe positions of phenotypes on the surface and to calculate changes in average phenotypes and concomitant changes in mean fitness. Lande's equation for change in average phenotype (1976, p. 317, Eq. 7) is (perhaps not surprisingly) similar to Wright's results for change in gene frequency per generation. Lande's analysis showed that the average phenotype of a population under natural selection (and given his two initial assumptions) is always in the direction of increase in mean fitness (i.e., *uphill* on the adaptive landscape), just as Wright had found for genotypes. Under certain circumstances, however, density-dependent selection can lead to a *decrease* in mean fitness.

Lande (1976) then considered the estimation of the role of drift, both in the development of trends within an adaptive zone and in phenotypic transformation resulting from shifts between adaptive zones (which, of course, are synonymous with adaptive peaks in Lande's terminology). Applying his equations to published data of examples of transformation in various taxa of fossil mammals, Lande (1976) consistently found that the transformations implied very weak intensities of selection, so weak that transformation by genetic drift alone could not be ruled out. He further considered the role of drift in changes between adaptive peaks—a topic we return to below, after considering recent work in patterns of phenotypic transformation.

Stasis and Transformation of Phenotypic Features: Recent Studies on Timing and Rates

Evolutionary biologists agree that the transformation of phenotypic structures on the whole represents adaptive modification through natural selection. Even according to the shifting balance theory, under which drift may enable a population to escape one peak for another (see below for further discussion), selection under most circumstances increases mean fitness, driving the population further up the peak, which by definition is a peak of optimality of adaptedness.

But we need to know more. We need to know when, and to what degree, phenotypic transformation takes place, and under what circumstances, during the history of any lineage of sexually reproducing organisms. We might assume, as a sort of null hypothesis, that selection and drift will keep a population oscillating in the vicinity of an adaptive peak. Such oscillation amounts to net evolutionary stability (as claimed by Wright, 1931, 1932; Lande, 1985, 1986; Newman et al., 1985)—provided that fitness values remain constant, which in general implies a constancy of environment. Environmental stability is generally cited as the major cause of *stabilizing selection*. However, several recent authors (e.g., Coope, 1979; Eldredge, 1985*b;* Vrba, 1985) have recognized that environmental change most often leads to habitat rearrangement. Organisms that can track familiar habitats through their spatial rearrangement (either through direct movement or through propagules) perceive the environmental change as, in fact, little or no change at all. Thus, in a very real sense, stabilizing selection is the norm when environments change as well as when they remain stable in any one local area for considerable periods of time. Stabilizing selection is likely to have been more important in the history of adaptive transformation than generally acknowledged in the past.

It should be noted, however, that Darwin (1859) and many successors, including Dobzhansky (1937*a*) and Simpson (1953), saw natural selection as a sufficiently powerful force for modification of modal phenotypes through time so that, given only sufficient variation, selection inevitably keeps improving adaptations even when the environment remains constant. In such formulations, there is usually seen to be a direct, if informally postulated, correlation between rate of transformation and rate or intensity of environmental change (whether biotic or abiotic, the source of the "selection forces" in Bock's, e.g., 1979, terminology).

Thus traditional Darwinism offers as a background null hypothesis the proposition that, all things being equal, we might anticipate directional adaptive change to be ongoing and progressive, occurring at more or less constant rates. Overall rate of change, in other words, is roughly equal to average rate of change when measured during any subinterval during the course of the history of a lineage. Yet, as we have seen, Wright's theory saw stability as the rule for much of the history of a local population: increase in mean fitness around an adaptive peak results in oscillating stasis; directional change comes only through peak shifts. Darwin himself, though he wrote of "insensibly graded series" of fossils forming sequences of transformational change through bodies of sedimentary rock, was aware that rates of change vary widely, not only among different lineages, but *within* lineages as well. Paleontologists reviewing the *Origin* (see Hull, 1973, for a compendium of such reviews) all noted that Darwin failed to acknowledge the great stability, the morphological conservatism, or lack of change, displayed by the majority of fossil species once they first appeared in the fossil record. By his sixth edition, Darwin (1872) had duly incorporated such stability in his discussion.

Gradualism is the term conventionally used to characterize slow, steady, progressive, intergradational evolutionary change. Though these adjectives are often included in characterizations of typical patterns of evolutionary change (Darwin, for example, clearly lumped all four in many of his passages), just as obviously the terms are not synonyms. "Gradual" rates can mean "intergradational," i.e., proceeding step by small incremental step. Most evolutionists are "gradualists" in this sense, the alternative being "saltationism," in which phenotypic transformation is held to occur in large, single steps. "Gradual" can also mean slow; or it can imply constant rates—or even a sense of progress, though the latter connotation is largely absent in modern evolutionary theory. Thus the term "gradual" is ambiguous, as not everyone has the same set of characteristics in mind when using the term.

Though Simpson (1970) has argued that Darwin was a gradualist only in the sense of "intergradational" or "graduated steps," most of Simpson's discussion of the historical sense of "gradualism" (mostly in a geological context) contrasts slow *and* small incremental steps of gradualism with the rapid and large-step events of "catastrophism." There is little doubt that Darwin also had the two senses of the term simultaneously in mind. The whole point of Darwin's discussions of geological time was to complete the analogy begun in his first chapter on domestic breeding: what animal husbandry could accomplish by artificial selection over generations would be magnified into the vast array of anatomical diversity, with the huge differences among organisms and the intricacies of their adaptations, given an earth whose age is measured in the hundreds of millions of years (a strong, if not utterly radical, proposition in the midnineteenth century).

Recent discussions have contrasted "phyletic gradualism" with "punctuated equilibria" (Eldredge, 1971; Eldredge and Gould, 1972; Gould and Eldredge, 1977; see Eldredge, 1985b, for a summary of the theory and its history). "Phyletic gradualism," to these authors, is the wholesale transformation of entire species (i.e., lineages in which sexual reproduction occurs among organisms within a reproductive community, but not, as a rule, with those belonging to other reproductive communities); the transformation is usually seen to be slow, steady, and intergradational. The more general term "phyletic evolution" refers to generation-by-generation modification of phenotypes and genotypes within a lineage, be that lineage a local population, an entire species, or, in some formulations, a taxon of higher rank.

In contrast, according to these authors, the bulk of the history of an entire species is best described as *stasis,* little or no directional change, but rather oscillations around some modal value for phenotypic features examined (Eldredge, 1971; Eldredge and Gould, 1972). "Punctuated equilibria" refers to a pattern, contrasted with phyletic gradualism, in which long periods of relative stasis are interrupted by relatively brief, hence relatively rapid, bursts of anatomical transformation—the "punctuations" of the "equilibria." Thus, these authors remained neo-Darwinian gradualists in the sense that the brief periods of relatively rapid change involved intergradational, rather than saltational, phenotypic transformation, presumably under the control of natural selection.

It is the pattern of anatomical change, rather than the details of its cause, which is of interest in this chapter. Eldredge (1971) and Eldredge and Gould (1972) argued that allopatric speciation in all likelihood underlies the production of the pattern. If speciation is defined as the formation of a descendant reproductive community (species) from an ancestral species (which continues to survive after the "speciation event"), the concentration of events of general adaptive change—i.e., involving nonreproductive (somatic) "economic" phenotypic attributes—at or near times of the origin of new reproductive communities raises serious theoretical issues bearing on the causality of adaptive change in evolution. These issues are addressed in ensuing chapters on speciation and the role played by species in nature in general and particularly in the (macro)evolutionary process.

For the purposes of this chapter, it is sufficient merely to discuss the pattern in terms strictly of transformational change—modifications of the phenotypic properties of organisms. Eldredge and Gould (1972) claimed that typical orders of magnitude for marine invertebrates would be between 5 to 10 million years of stasis (in long-lived species; many authors have noted that the fossil record tends to record the long-lived, widely dispersed species, to the detriment of our knowledge of species whose ranges are far more brief and geographically restricted). The issue is germane to a consideration of population genetics treatments of macroevolution, because some models have recently been developed that describe such "punctuated" patterns. We must ask: How common are patterns of "punctuated equilibria"? And what exactly are these patterns?

Systematists have relied (at least until the recent advent of molecular genetics) on comparative studies of organismic phenotypes for the characterization of species and their phylogenetic interrelationships. Thus all systematists are aware of what Hennig (1965) somewhat ponderously (if aptly) termed the "heterobathmy of synapomorphy." Synapomorphies are *shared derived features*, i.e., evolutionary novelties introduced at some point in the history of a taxon and inherited by all descendants in the same or further modified form. As we saw in Chap. 2, characters are introduced at various times in phylogeny and usually do not appear all at one time. The five digits of normal *Homo sapiens* hands and feet represent retention of the original tetrapod complement, a holdover from the Upper Paleozoic (some of the earliest tetrapods may have had additional digits, but the number five was "settled upon" early in tetrapod phylogeny). Mammalian hair was added somewhat later in phylogenetic history. And, of course, the expanded version of the primate brain characteristic of *Homo sapiens* came along still later. Thus novelties are distributed phylogenetically at "different depths" (heterobathmy). Depth can be viewed in terms of phylogenetic time or measured as breadth of distribution in different lineages: among vertebrates, four-leggedness is more widely distributed than hair, which is in turn more widely distributed than the anatomical configuration of the brain in *Homo sapiens*.

All this is to say that some characters will be expected to remain stable while others are changing, as a matter of course. Thus the issue of stasis vs. continuous, gradual change refers specifically to a limited subset of organismic phenotypic features: to those features that vary in the data set at hand, and in particular display a pattern of directional transformation. Thus we eliminate those features that show no evolutionary change within the lineage under study, removing a large bias that favors the impression of stasis, or morphological stability. We concentrate, instead, only on those features that undergo transformation: the problem is to understand the pattern of transformational change between two or more samples that appear to differ as a result of evolutionary modification.

Rigid stasis, of course, is rare for any phenotypic characteristic. Virtually all traits ever examined display some degree of intrapopulational or intraspecific variation.[1] In a study of an evolving lineage of the Middle Devonian trilobite *Phacops rana,* Eldredge (1972a) found an approximately constant width of variation in samples plotted against a multivariate vector (contrasting head size with number of lenses in the eye). The apparently linear trend showed a progressive increase of number of lenses in relation to head size, but showed some evidence, as well, for continued existence of variation in that relation through time.

Many studies reveal the entire spectrum of possibilities within the same data set: while most characters are stable, some show progressive change, while others display change concentrated in relatively brief episodes, interspersed with vastly longer periods of no change at all. Thus, in the trilobite example above, the trend towards lens increase per cephalon (head) size was abruptly reversed when the number of columns of lenses was (apparently relatively abruptly) reduced from 17 (the stable adult number for some 6 million years) to 15. More commonly, characters show patterns of oscillation around a mean, with no net directional change accruing; characters that do show a gradual, directional change commonly progress in a direction opposite to change when it occurs abruptly.

Stanley (1985) has pointed out that many of the published descriptions of long-term linear, phyletic transformation within lineages involve size changes. One of the examples analyzed by Lande (1976) from the fossil record was Gingerich's (1974, 1976) study of the Eocene mammal *Hyopsodus* (Fig. 3.1). Gingerich plotted the logarithm of surface area (i.e., $L \times W$) of the first lower molar M_1; he documented a gradual net increase in surface area of M_1 through a considerable segment of time—yet throughout there were several instances of small-scale directional changes *away* from the net direction of size increase. There were also several apparent bifurcations, with one branch showing progressive decrease in size, the other continuing the trend towards increase in molar (and hence presumably in overall body) size.

Gingerich, in the tradition of evolutionary paleontology ever since Darwin, prefers to recognize separate species as subdivisions of such evolving lineages. "Punctuationists," on the other hand, restrict the recognition of new species to lineages that arise as the result of splitting, i.e., true speciation in the biological sense. The new lineages are held to represent new reproductive communities, i.e., reproductively disjunct from the parental species. Changes—whether abrupt or linear—that do not appear to be the result of a true speciation process do not constitute a true example of punctuated equilibria. To a punctuationist, then, the issue is whether the phenotypic properties that differ between an ancestral species and its descendant arise relatively suddenly (just prior to, during, and just after the onset of reproductive isolation) or more broadly reflect patterns of change *within* the ancestral species gradually leading up to the morphology characteristic of the descendant species. The reader will appreciate that "species" and "speciation" mean considerably different things to "gradualists" and "punctuationists," a problem addressed more fully in Chap. 4, when we consider the nature of species.

It is also to be noted that punctuationists share a concern noted by the geneticist Richard Goldschmidt, whose notions of saltatory evolution via "hopeful monsters" arising from "systemic mutations" served as a foil for much of the rhetoric in the early documents of the modern synthesis (specifically, Dobzhansky, 1941; Mayr, 1942; Simpson, 1944). Goldschmidt (1940) based his theory on the observation that characters observed to be varying within biological species of the gypsy moth genus *Lymantria* did not appear to be the same as the phenotypic features that vary among arrays of closely related species of *Lymantria*. Thus, he concluded, there is no smooth adaptive continuum connecting within- and among-species variation.

Paleontologist Steven M. Stanley (especially 1979, 1985), a leading "punctuationist," has carefully examined the issue of frequency of punctuated vs. gradual patterns as documented in the paleontological literature. The slow rates of gradual transformation in most instances are insufficient to account for the accrued morphological changes ac-

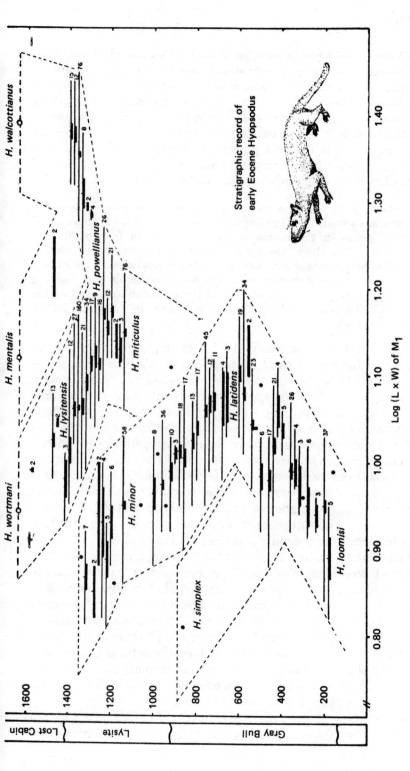

Figure 3.1 Gingerich's diagram of the "evolution of the early Eocene condylarth *Hyopsodus* in northern Wyoming." The figure plots the logarithm of the product of length and width of the first lower molar against the stratigraphic position of the sample. The range of variation is indicated by a horizontal line, standard error by a horizontal bar. (Redrawn from Gingerich, 1967, Fig. 5, p. 13)

69

tually observed between faunas; particularly because most examples involve simple size changes, such studies are not addressed to the actual patterns of change that distinguish ancestral from descendant species. Stanley (1985, p. 18) has put the case particularly well: noting that phyletic evolution is universal within lineages (given the nature of selection and drift acting on Mendelian populations), the question is: How important is it? Does phyletic evolution ever actually lead anywhere, i.e., underlie phenotypic change of significant magnitude? Stanley, discussing Gingerich's *Hyopsodus* work, says:

> Of relevance here is the fact that no branch in the phylogeny of *Hyopsodus* reconstructed by Gingerich moved beyond the confines of the original genus in the course of about 3.5 ma. In fact, within the *Hyopsodus* clade there was apparently little morphological evolution other than size change, which may have been punctuational. . . . Inasmuch as hundreds of new genera in many families of mammals were evolving during the persistence of the *Hyopsodus* clade, we can conclude that the sum total of evolution within *Hyopsodus* was trivial in the context of macroevolution.

Stanley's point is remarkably similar to Simpson's argument in 1944: at the observed rates of transformation, phyletic evolution is simply too slow to account for the observed phenotypic diversification that is going on in other lineages during any given interval of time. Recall that Lande (1976) found that published accounts of phyletic transformation require such weak selection coefficients that the possibility that the trends observed are the result of genetic drift cannot be ruled out. Simpson had restricted his remarks to taxa of higher categorical rank: even moderate rates of phyletic transformation are far too slow to account for the amount of phenotypic change characteristic of the origin of taxa of higher categorical rank, given that these taxa appear to evolve in rather brief intervals of time. The punctuationist—at least from the standpoint of patterns of phenotypic transformation—simply makes the point that even for species, anatomical differences between ancestor and descendant seldom appear to accrue through gradual phyletic evolution; rather, change appears concentrated in relatively rapid events. Regardless if the history of a species lineage reflects rigid stasis or (more commonly) oscillatory change at least in some phenotypic characteristics, or even if there is directional change throughout all or most of that history, the point is that seldom, if ever, does phyletic change lead to any major changes; meanwhile, major change typically is accruing in other lineages which are undergoing episodes of speciation: lineage splitting.

Though stasis—relative lack of significant phyletic change within species once they appear—has long been known to paleontologists, only since 1972 have there been a number of concerted efforts to document, and especially to quantify, the degree and commoness of stasis. Apart from the original examples and some earlier discussions and data (see Eldredge, 1971; Eldredge and Gould, 1972), there have been added a number of further examples. One technique to estimate stasis is simply to record the known stratigraphic ranges of species. Species in this sense can be viewed as "packages" of phenotypic properties; samples are considered conspecific through a stratigraphic interval so long as they simply remain recognizably the same, departing sufficiently little from their original morphology as developed in the earliest specimens that paleontologists regard the latest and all intervening specimens as conspecific. This informal, although not anecdotal, technique identifies entire faunas in which many species are seen to range through the entire stratigraphic interval. Thus, faunal lists, and especially charts graphically depicting stratigraphic ranges of species, constitute an informal measure of stasis in paleontological samples. In the Paleozoic, for example, faunas typically last from 5 to 10 million years. In the Hamilton Group (Middle Devonian), with over 500 named species of which at least 200 are valid, many species range throughout the known 6- to 8-million-year interval. Of these, few show more than minor oscillatory changes. Hallam (1976), in a survey of Jurassic bivalved mollusks, concluded that the average duration of a species is some 15 million years.

Sheldon (1987) has recently criticized the simple use of stratigraphic ranges of nominal species as a potentially biased estimator tending to exaggerate the prevalence of morphological stasis. Statistical (morphometric) analysis of quantitative characters avoids such bias. In a comprehensive study of Tertiary bivalves, Stanley and Yang (1987) analyzed a set of 24 variables for 19 lineages of Neogene bivalves, spanning time intervals of from 1 to 17 million years. One phase of their study entailed a comparison between Pliocene (4 million years old) samples and living populations of eight different species: they found that "...with minor exceptions, the distribution of morphological distances between 4 million years old and Recent populations resembled the distribution of distances between conspecific Recent populations" (Stanley and Yang, 1987, p. 113). For most lineages, Stanley and Yang found "weak and reversible trends," concluding that "evolution has followed a weak zigzag course, yielding only trivial net trends" and that "shape, as opposed to size, has been highly stable in bivalve evolution over millions of years and 10^6–10^7 generations" (Stanley and Yang, 1987, p. 113). For those who prefer visual evidence, Stanley and Yang offer two photographic figures documenting extraordinary conservatism within bivalve lineages over spans ranging from 4 to 17 million years (see Figs. 3.2 and 3.3).

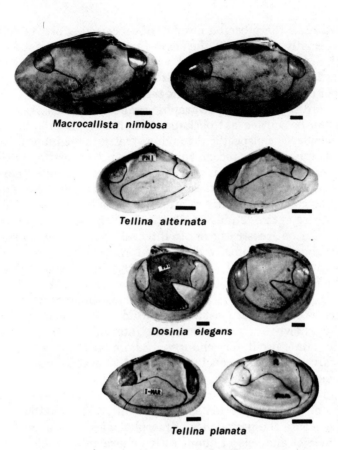

Macrocallista nimbosa

Tellina alternata

Dosinia elegans

Tellina planata

Figure 3.2 Comparison of 4-million-year old (*left*) and Recent (*right*) populations in four different bivalve species. Horizontal bar = 1 cm. (Adapted from Stanley and Yang, 1987, Fig. 4, p. 121; original illustration included statistical data pertaining to multivariate comparisons between samples)

Stanley (1985) has summarized many of the recent studies on patterns of stasis and transformation, producing a summary table reproduced here (Table 3.1); interestingly, his table supports prior estimates (see Eldredge, 1976) that, regardless of taxonomic affinity, marine organisms show far slower rates of phenotypic transformation than do terrestrial organisms.

Thus, stasis is a real phenomenon, especially if by stasis one means oscillatory variation, with no net directional change. Stasis has come to be accepted as a common and important evolutionary phenomenon by a wide range of paleontologists and evolutionary biologists, some of whom (e.g., Levinton, 1988) are otherwise staunchly opposed to the

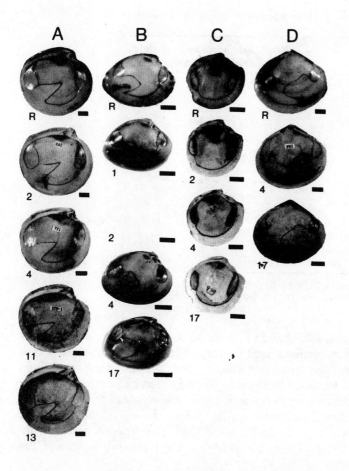

Figure 3.3 "Photographs of specimens belonging to four 'lineages' of bivalves. Numbers indicate age in millions of years. R = Recent; horizontal bar = 1 cm." (From Stanley and Yang, 1987, Fig. 11, p. 127)

theory of "punctuated equilibria." But even failing stasis, the sorts of directional evolution documented in some paleontological samples seem inadequate to account for the large-scale changes of macroevolution. Yet the converse is not thereby automatically established; we need to examine the evidence that phenotypic change really is concentrated in relatively rapid periods of time.

Punctuations and Transformational Change

Simpson was led to postulate rapid change in the origin of many taxa of relatively high categorical rank because (1) there was little or no

TABLE 3.1   Estimates of Mean Species Durations for a Variety of Biological Groups*

Biological group	Estimated mean species duration (millions of years)
Marine bivalves	11–14
Marine gastropods	10
	13.5
Benthic foraminifers	20–30
	> 20
Planktonic foraminifers	> 20
Freshwater fish	3
Beetles	> 2
Snakes	> 2
Mammals	> 1
	~2
Higher plants	> 8
	> 20
Bryophytes	≫ 20
Marine diatoms	25

*Based on Stanley (1985), Table 1, p. 16. Literature citations and methods of deriving estimates are included in Stanley's original table.

evidence of progressive change in a putative ancestor towards the new taxon, e.g., whales or bats, and (2) any of the possible ancestors (not known with precision for either whales or bats) in any case must have persisted in recognizable form after these groups had arisen. In other words, the origin of a higher taxon under the original formulation of quantum evolution involved a splitting from an ancestral stock that simply must have represented a rapid shift from the ancestral adaptations (morphology plus mode of life) to the new adaptations of the descendant taxon.

The theory of punctuated equilibria as originally and still most usefully construed makes the same requirements of any putative example as can be found in Simpson's discussions; the original examples (Eldredge, 1971; Eldredge and Gould, 1972) all involved *stratigraphic* (*i.e., temporal*) *overlap* between taxa interpreted as ancestral and descendant species. Such a requirement is logically necessary to postulate speciation as the underlying causal mechanism: speciation is the derivation of a daughter species from an ancestral species (alternatively, the splitting of ancestral species to yield two daughter species; see Chap. 4). For this reason, this stipulation of overlap in temporal ranges is an important aspect of the pattern of transformational change. It is also important because some paleontologists and geneticists (e.g., Lande, 1986) have claimed that punctuations do not typically reflect speciation, but actually represent a pattern of stepwise ("staircase," Stanley, 1985) change within single lineages. In other words, phyletic evolution may sometimes reflect a pattern of relative stasis interrupted by odd intervals of rapid transformation, rather than a pattern of progressive gradual change as traditionally envisioned. Micropaleontologist B. A. Malmgren and his colleagues (1983) have called this putative pattern "punctuated gradualism."

Abrupt changes within phyletic lineages—presumably, within entire species—are the sort of pattern underlying paleontologist Otto Schindewolf's (1950) notions of "typostrophic" saltationism, in which morphological transformations are seen to be saltatory interruptions of long periods of relative anatomical stability. Because Schindewolf applied his notions to species as well as to higher taxa, departing markedly from Darwinian gradualism, Simpson (1944) was especially concerned to refute his theory. Simpson saw similar patterns, denied that gaps between species were caused by anything other than hiatuses in the formation of the stratigraphic and fossil records, and claimed that gaps between higher taxa represent real evolutionary phenomena which could, however, be understood to result from a special concatenation of Darwinian "evolutionary determinants." Schindewolf, however vague his biological mechanisms were, saw abrupt, radical transformation of the phenotypes of organisms at all levels.

Yet care must be taken in interpreting any apparent pattern of abrupt phyletic change, with no stratigraphic overlap of ancestor and descendant. The fossil record is fraught with examples, making abrupt replacement of presumed ancestor by putative descendant more the rule than the exception. *Homo sapiens* abruptly replaces *Homo neanderthalensis* (some regard the two as but subspecies of a single species) in Europe about 34,000 years BP. Does this "event" represent (1) sudden transformation of ancestor into descendant, (2) a true event of speciation, in which descendant immediately annihilates its ancestor through competition (a model favored by some paleontologists, but which seems unlikely as a general rule), (3) a misinterpreted case of actual more gradual transformation (as some anthropologists, e.g., Wolpoff et al., 1984, still claim), or (4) an ecological or biogeographical event in which *H. sapiens* replaces *H. neanderthalensis,* either by direct extermination (more probable) or simply in expanding to take over vacated habitat space (less likely; see Tattersall, 1986; Stringer and Andrews, 1988)?

In the instance best known to me, taken from my own research and forming part of the original example of punctuated equilibria, there are three successive species (originally interpreted as subspecies: Eldredge, 1971; Eldredge and Gould, 1972) that succeed one another in Middle Devonian rocks in east central North America. There are no transitions; species occupy the continental interior seas for some millions of years, to be replaced abruptly by apparent descendants. The case, typical of many paleontological examples (including other lineages within the Hamilton Group), could involve (1) gradual, phyletic transformation (with the transitional forms simply missing from the record, which could happen if no sediments were preserved locally during the time interval in question) or (2) a sudden transformation reflecting saltationism, in the old parlance, or "punctuated gradualism," a form of neosaltationism preferred in some recent population genetics contributions (reviewed in the next section). It turns out that, in this particular Middle Devonian trilobite example (Fig. 3.4), there *was* a temporal gap at the critical place at both transitions. Perhaps as much as a million years is missing, and there is no way at all to judge just what went on. Fortunately, in this particular case, older samples from elsewhere (further east), at least in the case of the first two species, show unequivocally that the putative descendant species (*Phacops rana*) had already appeared as many as 2 million years *prior* to its first appearance in the Midwest habitat. Thus the staircase example in the Midwest reflects biogeographical replacement events, reflecting ecological rather than evolutionary history. Any study confined to only a portion of the range of species within a lineage is bound to produce similar misleading results. As Stanley (1985) concludes, the case for staircase evolution—for the ubiquity of "punctuated gradualism"—is suspect and weak.

As will be reviewed in greater detail in succeeding chapters, it is evident that there is no necessary relation between speciation and amount or nature of change in phenotypic properties, especially so-

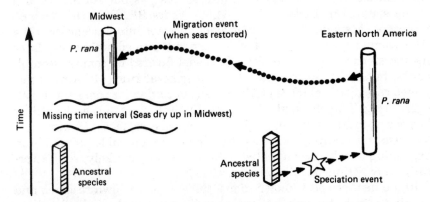

Figure 3.4 Diagram interpreting evolutionary history of the trilobite *Phacops rana* in midwestern and eastern North America. In the midwest, *P. rana* abruptly succeeds its presumed ancestor. *P. rana* appears earlier in rocks in the east and is interpreted to have arisen via speciation from the ancestor and to have spread later to the midwestern regions of the continent. For more detail, see text, and Eldredge, 1985*b*. (Modified from Eldredge, 1985*b*, p. 76)

matic ("economic") phenotypic attributes involved in nonreproductive functions and activities of organisms. This is to say that an entire spectrum of morphological divergence between closely related (as in parent-daughter) species is both expected and observed. Sibling species, for example, hardly differ at all morphologically; in other instances, more marked changes seem to be associated with speciation. In the published examples of punctuated changes known or suspected to be associated with lineage splitting (i.e., with speciation), the morphological changes are almost invariably rather minor in scope; typically, only a few features of the economic (nonreproductive) phenotype undergo modification. However, changes typically involve more than simple mean size and correlated shape changes. As an example, in one of the original examples of punctuated equilibria, simple change (reduction) in the number of vertical columns of lenses in the adult eye was documented in what were interpreted (Eldredge, 1972a) as a sequence of two successive speciation events. Williamson (1981) provides coordinate examples of morphological change associated with speciation in nine separate lineages undergoing speciation in response to geographical changes in a Pleistocene east African lake. Once again, the changes between ancestral and descendant species, while marked, are by no means great.

In the case of postulated phyletic events of relatively rapid change, once again we would expect there to be on theoretical grounds a spectrum of degrees of morphological change ranging from the very slight (as the most common) to the rather more profound. Goldschmidt's "hopeful monsters" (which were not based on empirically established actual examples) envisaged abrupt, saltatory transformations from one morphological configuration to another, as did Schindewolf's "typostrophism." As published in the paleontological literature, disruptions produced by apparently sudden events of morphological change (Stanley's "staircase" evolution) generally represent sudden changes in mean absolute size. The changes, while certainly statistically significant, generally represent no large departure in morphological configuration (shape changes, if they occur, usually are simple allometric correlates of size change). As in cases of apparent lineage splitting, the large majority of examples of such "punctuations" exhibit rather minor amounts of morphological change.

Absolute duration of punctuation events is also critical to any modeling of underlying causal processes involved in their production. True saltation theories, such as those of Goldschmidt and Schindewolf, postulate virtual overnight change. Whatever the mechanism, mutations (including, as most commonly cited, chromosomal rearrangements) lie at the heart of most such speculative theories. Most recently, a number of authors have proposed that relatively minor changes in the regulatory apparatus (genes that control the expression of so-called structural genes, i.e., those that code for particular enzyme products) may produce cascading effects in the ontogenetic development of organisms; by the time ontogeny is complete, the adult morphology may be rather radically altered. In any case, a single, or at most a few, generations are usually supposed to be involved in any true case of saltation.

Proponents of punctuated equilibria have noted the difficulties attached to documenting actual transitions between ancestor and descendant. As Darwin (1859), Dobzhansky (1937a), and especially Simpson (1944) pointed out, the actual evidence for periods of rapid evolution lies in the *absence* of samples of morphologically variable or intermediate organisms. In particular, the model of *peripatric speciation* (Mayr, 1954, followed closely by Eldredge, 1971; Eldredge and Gould, 1972, in the early formulation of punctuated equilibria) sees new species arising as isolates on the periphery of the ancestral species' range; population size and other factors conspire to reduce the probability of finding such intermediates in the fossil record in the early throes of the speciation process. Nonetheless, intermediate populations (Eldredge, 1972a) were postulated in the original trilobite example used to support the idea of punctuated equilibria. Rule-of-thumb estimates have led to the generalization that anywhere from 5000 to 50,000 years may be involved in such speciation events. This is indeed brief when compared with the 1- to 10-million-year average duration of species once established (depending on the taxon; see Table 3.1); hence the term "punctuated." Yet, from the standpoint of genetics, these rates are moderate to slow; speciation is known to occur much more quickly in some instances and circumstances.

In the case of putative "staircase" evolution, estimates of rate likewise vary. The notion of "bottlenecks," where species are imagined to be greatly reduced in numbers, creating the opportunity for rapid genetic and phenotypic change lasting but a few thousands of years, has occasionally been used to account for brief spurts of rapid phyletic evolution interrupting much longer periods of slower phyletic change. More detailed consideration of the conditions and rates of genetic and phenotypic change in phyletic evolution can be found in the "peak shift" models of Wright, Lande, and other population geneticists.

Population Genetics and Macroevolution II.
Peak Shifts and Punctuated Patterns

Wright (1982, 1988) has pointed out that his shifting balance theory anticipated the pattern of stasis and relatively rapid change that underlies the notion of punctuated equilibria. Indeed, it was these elements of Wright's model that attracted Simpson's attention. The theory of punctuated equilibria relates the pattern of stasis and change to within- and among-species-level phenomena, i.e., more nearly to the level which Wright originally addressed, rather than strictly to the higher taxa to which Simpson restricted his quantum evolution model. Yet Mayr (1982b) is undoubtedly correct in asserting that Wright's models have always been directed to "vertical evolution," i.e., within-species phyletic evolution (however nonlinear the patterns might be) rather than to speciation per se. Simpson likewise regarded speciation as relatively minor and of no particular importance in macroevolution.

Geneticists extending the Wright-Simpson analysis to encompass patterns of punctuated change likewise discount the possible connection of such patterns with true speciation (i.e., where lineage splitting is involved). As we have already noted, Lande (1986) argues that most punctuated patterns in fact reflect what Stanley (1985) has termed staircase evolution: phyletic progression marked by long periods of relative conservatism (stasis, fluctuations, or slow directional phyletic modification), "punctuated" on occasion by rapid state changes. Such a visualization fits Simpson's (1953, p. 389) modified conceptualization of quantum evolution as a "special, more or less extreme and limiting case of phyletic evolution."

Geneticists utilizing Wright's adaptive landscape imagery naturally see phenotypic transformation as a matter of shift between two peaks of mean fitness on the adaptive landscape. Though the usual language used ("population") generally connotes one of several subgroups within a species, what is intended, at least in the recent literature—and presumably in Wright's (1982) remarks about the similarities between his shifting balance theory and punctuated equilibria—is that entire lineages, i.e., entire species, undergo such shifts, without branching.

Lande (1985, 1986), Newman et al. (1985), and other geneticists as well have recently begun to address explicitly patterns of punctuated change (Fig. 3.5). Though such patterns by definition must be consistent with population-level genetic processes, their importance as a general pattern of evolutionary phenotypic transformation had not been anticipated (predicted) by general evolutionary genetic theory, despite the availability of the shifting balance theory since the early 1930s.[2] Now that the patterns have been established as sufficiently general, geneticists have become concerned to describe them with equations—specifically diffusion equations that describe patterns of phenotypic and genotypic transformation on Wright's adaptive topography in the basic manner discussed earlier in this chapter.

Selection always acts to drive a population up an adaptive peak of

Mean character $\bar{x}$

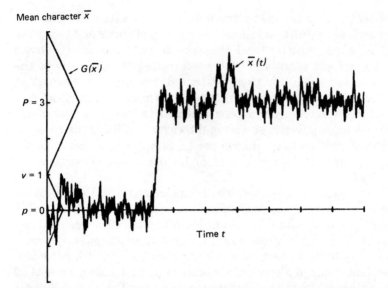

Figure 3.5 "Punctuated shifting equilibria" of Newman, et al. (1985). The diagram also serves to illustrate what other authors have called "stepwise" or "staircase" evolution, and approximates the "punctuated gradualism" of still other authors. The original caption of this diagram is as follows: "Punctuated equilibria in a numerical solution of the discrete time equation $\dot{x}(t+1) - x(t) = G'(\bar{x}(t)) + sw_t$. The landscape G has a lower peak at $\bar{x} = 0$, a valley at $\dot{x} = 1$ and a higher peak at $\dot{x} = 3$; its slope, G', takes only the values $+0.01$ or -0.01. w_t represents the sign of random variables, s their magnitude. For each t, w_t is independently $+1$ or -1 with equal probability; $s = 0.07$. The jagged line plots $x(t)$ for 5000 time units. As theory predicts, during the transition between peaks, $\dot{x}$ moves from 0 to 1 as if the direction of natural selection were reversed, that is, at the same speed that $\dot{x}$ moves by natural selection from 1 to 3." (Redrawn from Newman et al., 1985, Fig. 1, p. 400)

mean fitness (assuming constancy of fitness): Wright's original solution confirmed by Lande (1976) for polygenic phenotypic characters. Investigating how a population could, under such circumstances, leave one peak and gain another, both Lande (1985) and Newman et al. (1985) found that drift, working against selection, can send a population down a slope—the population genetics counterpart to Simpson's suggestion of an "inadaptive phase," in which original adaptations are lost in the first phase of his tripartite model of "quantum evolution." Moreover, such downward, drift-induced progression can be rapid; indeed, as Newman et al. suggest, it is only when drift is rapid that the effects of selection can be overcome.

The models of both Lande and Newman et al. further show that, regardless of population size, the time spent in the valley between peaks is always very brief. And both analyses confirm the standard expectation that once the slope of the second adaptive peak is reached, selection rapidly drives the population uphill. The models, utilizing equations developed to describe diffusion processes, show that the same results obtain regardless of population size. However, punctuational events are less frequent the larger the populations, as the probability that drift will be able to counteract the effects of selection decreases as population size increases. The events still happen, but they are relatively more rare, with intervening periods of stasis correspondingly proportionately still longer, the bigger the population. And it is the large populations that are sampled more readily in the fossil record.

Newman et al. (1985) further point out that gradual evolution is possible given a gradual shift in position of adaptive peaks, i.e., in fitness values, occasioned by environmental change. Superimposing their model on such a gradually changing adaptive landscape yields a pattern of "punctuated shifting equilibria" (Newman et al., 1985, p. 400). Thus punctuations are found to be possible even in the context of gradual phyletic change: populations may track a moving peak, occasionally shifting abruptly from that peak to another in the field. The model is strongly reminiscent of the qualitative picture developed by Simpson (1944, 1953), once again, with the proviso that Simpson had higher taxa (macroevolution, or his "megaevolution") particularly in mind. The models developed independently by Newman et al. (1985) and Lande (1985) are more general in that they posit patterns of abrupt transformation of phenotypic characters of unspecified magnitude.

Thus in recent years population genetics, particularly in the work of Lande, has moved to analyze patterns of phenotypic transformation in explicit detail. In addition to standard neo-Darwinian considerations of smooth, continuous, intergradational, as well as constant and rather slow, rates (i.e., the amalgam of attributes usually summarized as "gradual" transformation through time), geneticists have recently begun to consider the possibility that patterns of abrupt punctuational change are intergradational but much more rapid than vastly longer periods of either relative stasis or very slow change.

It remains a generalization acceptable to virtually all evolutionary biologists that there is a spectrum of rates, and of constancy of those rates, of phenotypic change in the evolutionary process. However, especially in the consideration of transformations of sufficiently great magnitude to fall under the informal rubric of "macroevolution," a consensus seems to be emerging that unusually rapid rates, concentrated in relatively brief episodes or bursts, are the norm rather than the exception. As Simpson, and later Stanley, have been arguing, the pattern of sudden appearance of highly derived (phenotypically modified) taxa admits of no other conclusion.

Simpson's models, based on a qualitative application of Wright's quantitative genetics, especially his utilization of adaptive landscape imagery in the formulation of his shifting balance theory, focused on macroevolution. But, as we have just seen, recent work in population genetics modeling in effect generalizes, as well as quantifies, Simpson's models, developing analytic descriptions of punctuated patterns that hold for all manner of population sizes and (presumably) degree of anatomical change. The theory of punctuated equilibria, explicitly based on speciation theory, also represented a scaling down of the pattern and phenomena Simpson addressed in his theory of quantum evolution (at least in its original version). Some biologists (including myself) are persuaded that the bulk of change—be it adaptive or heavily influenced as well by genetic drift—is concentrated in episodes of speciation. But, more generally, it seems that a consensus has emerged that punctuated patterns of phenotypic transformation can and do occur; indeed, they seem to be the rule in evolution.

Thus the biological context of adaptive stasis and transformation appears to be coming into somewhat sharper focus. How such generalized models (such as the models of Lande and other geneticists, as well as the theory of punctuated equilibria, which deal in the main with small-scale patterns of change) can be seen to relate to the question of large-scale adaptive transformation will emerge in later segments of this book, especially after a consideration of the nature of species, higher taxa, and other large-scale biological entities. For the moment, the concern in this chapter remains with models of neo-Darwinian processes and the production of patterns of adaptive transformation.

The Red Queen

Van Valen's (1973) "Red Queen hypothesis" was advanced as a conjecture to explain his "law of constant extinction," newly formulated in that same paper. Van Valen (1973) presented a series of taxonomic survivorship curves for some 43 different taxa (Fig. 3.6). The curves simply plot the "proportion of the original sample [i.e., a subgroup of some larger taxon] that survive for various intervals" (Van Valen, 1973, p. 1). A number of authors have criticized the compilation of the survivorship curves themselves. And McCune (1982, p. 610) has pointed out that even if the curves *are* linear, "constant extinction rates cannot be deduced from Van Valen's survivorship curves." The real implication of such curves, she argues, is that "probability of extinction of a taxon is independent of its duration."

The Red Queen hypothesis accounts for the supposed constancy of extinction rates of subtaxa within a monophyletic clade (e.g., of genera within a family) by constructing a model that sees other taxa (spe-

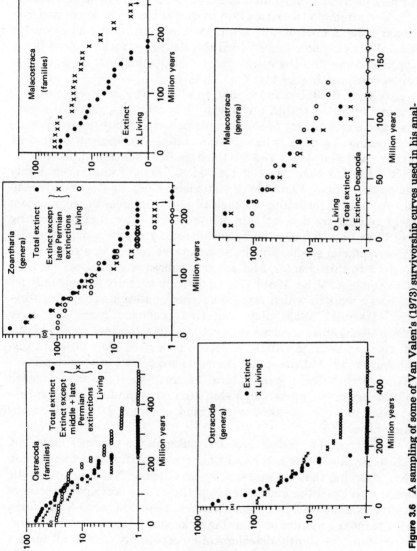

Figure 3.6 A sampling of some of Van Valen's (1973) survivorship curves used in his analysis of extinction rates and his discussion of the Red Queen hypothesis. (Redrawn from Van Valen, 1973, Fig. 3, p. 4)

cifically species) as the most important factor in the evolutionary environment of any given, focal species. Utilizing the imagery of the adaptive landscape, Van Valen (1973, p. 17) considers together "the various species in an adaptive zone."[3] Because the Red Queen model, utilizing the imagery of the adaptive landscape, attempts to address the conditions and typical rates of evolutionary transformation, and in particular attempts to extrapolate from short-term to long-term evolutionary change, its details are important despite the questionable status of the phenomena for which the Red Queen was originally developed and the dubious attribution of niches and adaptive zones to taxa (species and higher taxa).

Van Valen (1973) concluded that, in view of the putative constancy of extinction rates within any given "homogeneous group of organisms," the environment of the organisms within that group must be deteriorating at a more or less constant rate—a generalization that he characterized as a "law." Though the data from which he inferred constancy of extinction rates pertained to actual (and presumably monophyletic) taxa, Van Valen's statement of his "law" was more general, explicitly including ecologically comparable organisms *not* closely related by descent (his example was mice and fruit-eating flies). Thus Van Valen, at base, considered a cross-genealogical situation: (sympatric) species within an "adaptive zone." As already noted in Note 3 in this chapter, and as some subsequent analysts have already seen (e.g., Vrba, 1988), this suggestion is really tenable only for local ecosystems in which representative populations of species ("avatars," Damuth, 1985) play concerted economic roles, i.e., have "niches." That entire species, as a rule, are not confined to single ecosystems, and because different species, as a rule, have different distributions, such that the same species do not occur together in all ecosystems within their geographical ranges, the relevance of such evolutionary modeling as Van Valen's to understanding long-term evolutionary histories of entire species (and, of course, larger-scale taxa) is not entirely clear.

Nonetheless, the Red Queen and subsequent versions have had much to say about the rates and timing of evolutionary change. Van Valen, claiming that his model accommodates both abiotic and biotic change, developed the Red Queen hypothesis as a descriptive motor of adaptive change. Holding the abiotic regime constant, Van Valen (1973) painted a picture of "running to keep in place"—the "effective" environment, constantly deteriorating, perpetually forcing all species in the system to keep undergoing modification merely to retain their original level of adaptedness. Thus, in this particular visualization of biotic nature, evolutionary modification of all species is inevitable and rather constant. Vrba (1980) has pointed out that the Red Queen is the very personification of evolutionary gradualism.

The Red Queen assumes tight interconnectedness, or, in ecological parlance, a high level of *accommodation* that interlinks the species within the system. In particular, Van Valen (1973) specified a "zero-sum" assumption, in which all evolutionary change (increase in fitness) for any one species is counterbalanced *exactly* by negative pressures on one or more different species within the evolving system. Assuming high interconnectedness among species, evolutionary improvement for one species suggested to Van Valen that some other species must become correspondingly less well adapted: if the improvement were in the utilization of a food resource shared with a second species, the second species would undergo a decrease in fitness, as would, of course, the food resource species. Thus species emerge, under the Red Queen, as being in a state of constant flux; and species interconnected ecologically form systems that almost resemble evolutionary perpetual motion machines. Disruptions of the constant motor of evolutionary change arise solely from perturbations, especially those arising from the abiotic environment.

Some years later, Stenseth and Maynard Smith (1984) reexamined the Red Queen explicitly in an ecosystem context. They were concerned to develop a model of ecosystem coevolution that describes "the whole community, and not subsets of species within it." It should, further, describe "both the densities of genetically constant species, and evolutionary changes in those species," as well as "how the number and types of species in the community change." It is clear that Stenseth and Maynard Smith were examining "avatars," the useful term for local populations of conspecifics playing a concerted, specifiable economic role in a local ecosystem; it is such units, not species per se, that in fact have ecological "niches." We have already encountered the confusion between concepts of adaptive peaks and zones, on the one hand, and ecological niches on the other. Some authors treat adaptive peaks as though they are niches. Yet it is by no means clear, in the models of (mean) genetic fitness, as well as in Lande's phenotypic models utilizing the imagery of the adaptive landscape, that "increase in mean fitness" is to be construed as "improvement in niche utilization."

Indeed, Stenseth and Maynard Smith conceptually divorce "ecological advantage" from changes in *lag load*. In an attempt to provide a more precise formulation of distance of a population from its local adaptive peak, they utilize Maynard Smith's own earlier concept of evolutionary lag load. Lag load is defined as the difference between the fittest possible genotype to the *present* environment (including mutations as yet unrealized) ($\hat{W}$) and present mean fitness $\overline{W}$, divided by $\hat{W}$ simply to normalize. Any change in Van Valen's "effective environment" amounts to a change in the location of the peak, automatically implying a change in value of $\hat{W}$; as Stenseth and Maynard Smith report, assuming that most species are fairly close to their adaptive peaks, most shifts in peak positions will probably be away from $\overline{W}$, and hence will result in an increase in lag load. In their model, lag load can increase even if there is a temporary ecological advantage gained by a species (as measured by an increase of numbers of organisms in the local population).

Stenseth and Maynard Smith derive a series of equations that address the fates of mean lag load (of species in general within the system) as well as the number of species present in the system (as affected by speciation and extinction). Of the possible solutions to the equations under a variety of parameter values, they conclude that only two possibilities are realistic. One conforms closely to Van Valen's original Red Queen, even if the assumption of "zero sum" is ignored (Stenseth and Maynard Smith reject it as unrealistic), but provided that the level of biotic accommodation is high within a local ecosystem. If not—if, instead, there is rather little interspecific interaction within the ecosystem—then Stenseth and Maynard Smith conclude that it is the abiotic, physical environment that essentially drives evolution. In this, the second possibility, when there is no abiotic environmental change, evolution essentially grinds to a halt. Species "are expected to remain phenotypically fairly constant for extensive periods" (Stenseth and Smith, 1984, p. 878). Evolutionary change is expected to occur in bursts "associated with, and caused by, major changes in the physical environment." There are consequences for species number and extinction rates within ecosystems, as well.

While they acknowledge that "it is tempting to suggest that" the contrast between the Red Queen and Stationary models corresponds to the contrast between gradualism and a "stasis plus punctuation interpretation of the fossil record," Stenseth and Maynard Smith (1984), for unspecified reasons, write that they "cannot support this interpretation strongly." Yet they do maintain that "it is relevant that a strictly Darwinian model, in which evolutionary changes occur because of intrapopulational selection, can lead either to continual change or to stasis depending on the nature of the ecological and evolutionary interactions between species."

Vrba (1988) has pointed out that Stenseth and Maynard Smith have confused the sorts of processes that affect local populations of species integrated into local ecosystems with those that affect the phylogenetic histories of entire species. Within such local populations, there are processes of stasis and change in gene content and frequency, as well as origin and disappearance (through migration and actual organismic death) of the local populations. These are not the same as (1) accrual of concerted, specieswide genetic change or (2) speciation and true species extinction. It becomes clear that Van Valen's model, if assumed plausible as developed for local populations within ecosystems, cannot facilely be extrapolated to the phylogenetic (species) level. Vrba (1988) is at pains to discuss the care that must be taken to bridge the manifest lack of congruence between ecological and phylogenetic models. These issues are discussed in greater detail in ensuing chapters, when the nature of entities—especially species—and the actual roles they play in nature are examined.

Yet there *is* a connection between Van Valen's Red Queen model, on the one hand, and truly phylogenetic patterns of stasis and change on the other, a connection that becomes evident when Wright's (1931, 1932) imagery of species distributed in quasi-isolated "colonies" is added to Van Valen's picture. As Wright argued, each colony has a quasi-autonomous evolutionary history; it is through the simultaneous and independent exploration of gene combinations within such local colonies that a species as a whole is able more readily to locate the higher peaks in the adaptive landscape, a vital part of Wright's shifting balance theory. Put in terms of the Red Queen, each local population within a given species is a part of a local ecosystem, and each local ecosystem differs in some respects from all others. Under the Red Queen, in highly accommodated ecosystems, each local population does indeed have an evolutionary history that may well involve continuous (and appreciable) genetic and phenotypic change.

However, the history of each local population, following Wright, is ordinarily expected to differ from the histories of conspecific populations in other ecosystems. Selection forces—to use Bock's (1979) term—most likely differ somewhat from one local ecosystem to another; genetic drift histories are even more certain to differ from one local population to the next. Also—and as stressed by Futuyma (1987) and reviewed more extensively in later chapters—within-population evolutionary change is inherently unstable and ephemeral, as the fate of local populations is often extinction or amalgamation with other populations. And thus there should be no net concerted specieswide change accumulating on a phylogenetic basis. Ironically, the Red Queen, when added to Wright's depiction of the structure of single species in nature, is probably the best single theoretical reason to expect net, specieswide stasis: geographically based variability that is seldom cumulatively and significantly modified in any particular direction throughout the subsequent history of an entire species.

There is a final corollary to this discussion: We would expect that most published accounts documenting "phyletic gradualism"—where there appears to be some (directional) accrual of phenotypic change within a lineage through time—would be restricted to local, quasi-autonomous populations, found in rather limited geographical areas. Such is the case, for example, in Gingerich's (e.g., 1976) examples, all of which come from the Bighorn Basin (despite the fact that all the taxa are known to occur in other intermontane basins as well). It is true, also, of the eight trilobite lineages discussed by Sheldon (1987), all of which come from the Builth Inlier, a rather restricted area in Wales. A further test of this generalization awaits study of the histories of populations of a single species in different ecosystems, always a difficulty because of problems in establishing contemporaneity between far-flung samples.

The models of Van Valen and Stenseth and Maynard Smith are valuable and instructive in part simply because they explicitly address (parts of) more than one species at a single time. Evolutionary theory has historically focused on breeding populations, species, and monophyletic taxa. It has been especially concerned with the fates of adaptations. To be sure, most organismic adaptations are concerned with the *economic* activities of organisms. Yet, as is apparent from the Red Queen discussion above, there is need for an even sharper picture of the actual nature of such entities as species and monophyletic taxa, the better to analyze their role in the evolutionary process, including the history of phenotypic adaptive change. And we need to go beyond the work of Van Valen, Stenseth and Maynard Smith, and others to incorporate the organization of large-scale ecological systems into the evolutionary picture.

In sum, the status of microevolutionary modeling of macroevolutionary change has taken some interesting turns in recent years. Older models assumed virtual constancy of rates of genotypic and phenotypic change. Exceptions—such as Simpson's early version of "quantum evolution"—were rooted in the empirical observation of relatively sudden appearances of large-scale phenotypic change, implying periods of rapid change marking the appearance of major innovations. And Sewall Wright's "shifting balance theory," based as it was on a compelling picture of species fragmented into "semi-isolated colonies," has provided the basis of much of the more recent progressive work in realistic evolutionary models. More recent discussion of the great phenotypic stability exhibited by the majority of species known over segments of geological time measured in the millions of years has reinforced such notions of variation in rate, so that now rapid change followed by longer periods of relative evolutionary stability—*non*change—seems the norm for many different taxa. That mathematically inclined geneticists are now prompted to model such patterns of adaptive change is a definite step forward in bringing closer together the typical, recurrent patterns in the evolutionary history of life with our ideas on how the evolutionary process actually works.

Notes to Chapter 3

1. The modern synthesis placed great emphasis on intrapopulational and intraspecific (particularly geographical) variation. Such emphasis to some extent reflects a theoretical concern, i.e., that within-species adaptive morphological differentiation serves as a precursor to among-species morphological differences, forming a continuum disrupted only by reproductive isolation; it appears (at least to me) that degree and ubiquity of within-species variation has been commonly and routinely exaggerated over the past 50 years. Nonetheless, such variation obviously does occur in all samples of fossil and Recent organisms.

2. Though punctuated patterns, whether or not entailing lineage splitting (speciation), did not arise as a general prediction from standard neo-Darwinian evolutionary theory over the past 50 years, geneticists could hardly be faulted for not being informed of the pattern by paleontologists, who are in by far the best position to establish the generality of the pattern.

3. As will be discussed in greater detail in later chapters, there are strong reasons *not* to see species (or higher taxa) as *wholes* acting as parts of ecosystems. Thus species as entire entities do not possess "niches," nor can they be said to occupy "adaptive peaks" or "adaptive zones." If, however, the reader takes Van Valen's (1973) discussion to read "local populations of species"—which are, of course, parts of local ecosystems—the model can be seen to address realistically aspects of biological organization in nature. This is precisely the sense, for example, in which Stenseth and Maynard Smith (1984) take the Red Queen and related models.

Chapter 4

Species,
Speciation,
and Transformational
Stasis and Change

One hundred and thirty years after the publication of Darwin's *On the Origin of Species,* there is still substantial, even profound, disagreement and confusion about the very nature of *species.* Yet it is obvious that we need a clear idea of what species are before we can speak of the manner of their evolutionary origin. Not that there has been no progress in the debate on species since Darwin's day; the prime goal of this chapter is to review the current status of the issue of species *ontology* (i.e., what species *are*). Such a review permits a classification of speciation mechanisms, which leads directly to a consideration of the relation between speciation (the origin of new species) and the more general issue of the transformation of phenotypic organismic features.

In a sense, the fundamental issue in the ongoing debate about the nature of species seems to be merely a matter of emphasis: most biologists would agree that, at least within the same sex, members of a "species" tend to resemble one another more than they do members of other "species." So the notion of species has something to do with phenotypic similarity shared by some organisms that sets them apart from other collections of likewise similar organisms. Such a definition dominates, for example, textbooks in introductory biology.

Yet it is equally clear that sexually reproducing organisms draw mates from a community that is strictly limited in scope: there is a community of organisms within which suitable mates can be found and beyond which successful mating cannot occur. Moreover, it is the replication of genes underlying the reproductive process that causes

organisms to resemble their parents and that further leads to maintenance of phenotypic similarity among communities of organisms—
"species." Thus the mating capabilities of sexual organisms is strongly
connected with any idea of what species might be and might even be
seen to be a primary criterion.

Locally (i.e., *sympatrically,* meaning living at the same time and
place), sexually reproducing organisms as the overwhelming rule fall
into clear-cut morphological groups. Mating, when it occurs, is restricted solely to members of that group, which are seen to be distinguished generally by a number of morphological features *some of
which pertain to reproduction, others of which pertain to nonreproductive aspects of the organisms' biology.* As a rule, there is close
agreement between species as clusters of reproducing organisms and
as clusters of phenotypically similar organisms. It is to be noted, however, that sexually reproducing animals in general display greater degree of concordance between groups delineated by overall phenotypic
similarity and those recognized by reproductive behavior than plants
might show. In particular, many groups of plants appear morphologically distinct, but hybridize regularly and freely with other "species"
recognized on morphological grounds. Thus botanists have historically
resisted the movement (so common in animal-oriented evolutionary
biology of the past 50 years) to recognize "species" *primarily* as reproductive communities (the "biological species concept"—see below).

While the sympatric case generally develops the greatest degree of
agreement between species conceptualized as morphologically distinct
and differentiated groups of organisms and species seen as reproductive communities, there are further exceptions to this generalization.
So-called *sibling species* are an instructive case in point. Not to be confused with "sister species" in phylogenetic systematics (see Chap. 5),
sibling species consist of sympatric organisms that appear to form a
single, coherent group, based on the assessment of overall morphological similarity, but on closer inspection prove to comprise two (or even
more) separate reproductive communities. In other words, the slight
phenotypic differences between sibling species pertain especially—
perhaps even solely—to aspects of their reproductive biology. Morphologically, perhaps even ecologically, sibling species may be identical,
or at least so similar that their status as separate breeding communities may at first be overlooked.

It is when organisms from different places (i.e., *allopatric*) and different times (sometimes called *allochronic*) are compared that problems begin to become compounded. Deciding whether to call such
allochronic or allopatric populations members of the same species or of
two or more separate species is not, of course, merely a matter of
methodological protocol. Rather, the conceptual difficulties inherent

in the ontology of species as developed so far in biology are simply pushed to the limit. Thus, some biologists, believing that joint reproductive community status can be inferred for allopatric populations, assign two rather well (morphologically) differentiated populations to the same species. In contrast, however, many systematists would prefer to recognize well-differentiated allopatric populations as separate "species," even if there is evidence that those allopatric populations retain the capacity for interbreeding. As reviewed below, and further in Chap. 6, such disagreement hinges on what biologists think species fundamentally *are*, i.e., whether they see species primarily as reproductive communities or as groups of organisms united first and foremost by shared possession of phenotypic properties.

Reproductive and Economic Phenotypic Properties

The distinction between reproductive and economic phenotypic properties lies at the heart of biological controversy over the nature of species. Economic attributes are those involved with the differentiation, growth, and maintenance of the soma (the *nonreproductive* aspects of the phenotype). Reproductive attributes involve the germ-line cells, tissues, and organs, as well as aspects of the soma (and associated physiologies and behaviors) concerned in whole or in part with reproduction.

We note right away that there are several broad areas of overlap between these two categories. Prokaryotic microorganisms (bacteria) show little differentiation (anatomically and physiologically) between the two sets of activities, while multicellular organisms, with the germ line well differentiated from the soma, show the clearest distinction. Further, as Darwin (1871) was probably the first to discuss with clarity, some aspects of organismic phenotypes are involved in more than one function; the distinction is most ambiguous, as Darwin noted, in some "secondary sexual characteristics," a topic to which we return below in conjunction with a consideration of Paterson's (e.g., 1985) concept of "species mate recognition systems." And, finally, it is clear that even primary sexual organs themselves are parts of the soma, and that reproduction requires expenditure of energy. Then, too, gonadal hormonal secretions circulating within a mammalian body profoundly influence many aspects of physiology and behavior not geared directly, or primarily, to reproduction. Thus in drawing a distinction between two broad categories of organismic phenotypic properties, there is no implication that anatomically the two are wholly isolated. The distinction between reproductive and economic aspects of the phenotype is reminiscent of, but strictly speaking not the same as, Weismann's distinction between the germ line and the soma. The two differ primarily in that reproductive adaptations subject to sexual selection entail elements (such as primary sex organs) that are themselves aspects of the soma.

Though the two sets of features are complexly interrelated, the distinction between reproductive and economic (matter-energy) aspects of organismic phenotypes is well worth drawing, particularly when we recall that it is the transformation of organismic phenotypic properties that formed the original (and still central) question in evolutionary biology. But even beyond the confines of evolutionary biology, physiologists have also found the distinction worthwhile, noting that of all categories of physiological function, only reproduction is not essential to the continued existence of an individual organism. Reproduction is a thing apart from the ongoing processes crucial to continued somatic survival (i.e., respiration, excretion, etc.).

But it is Darwin's argument that *natural selection* is distinct from *sexual selection* that highlights the importance of distinguishing the two categories of organismic phenotypic properties in an evolutionary context. Darwin supposed that, in a world of finite resources, phenotypic variation among organisms (within a reproductive community) would confer advantages to some organisms over others: some would be faster, or more efficient foragers, etc. The important causal link in Darwin's notion of natural selection is that, on average, the advantage an organism might have over some others within a local population might well be expected to have a side effect on successful reproduction: on average, Darwin postulated, the organisms thriving economically will tend to fare better reproductively as well. And, because offspring tend to resemble their parents, the reproductive advantage gained by those parents with economic advantages will result in a shift in succeeding populations towards more organisms with the traits that confer such economic success.

The concept of *fitness* in modern population genetics merges a notion of economic success directly with reproductive success. "Fitness," a connotation of robusticity in Darwin's day, is now defined as "probability of reproductive success"—taken as a reflection of relative economic success, among other factors. But it is vital, for a clear grasp of the causality involved, to see the matter more as Darwin originally did: natural selection is the influence of relative economic success (as a statistical side effect) on the reproductive success of organisms.

Thus, in Darwin's world view, there was a need to recognize another category of reproductive success: that arising through the "advantage which certain individuals have over other individuals of the same sex and species, in exclusive relation to reproduction" (Darwin, 1871, p. 256). In other words, some organisms, by dint of some combination of behavioral, morphological, and physiological characteristics, are simply better at reproducing than are others. It is not because they are faster runners or more efficient foragers: they are simply better at finding mates and reproducing. These traits, too, of course are "selected," as they are preferentially handed down to succeeding generations. As some biologists have pointed out, it is situations in which conflicts arise that the difference between two selective regimes is most clearly seen, as when the sexual selection underlying male peacock display morphology and behavior conflicts with long-term survival chances of such males, who are expected to be more attractive prey items than the duller females. Many male song birds lose their bright breeding plumage, becoming like the more cryptic females, after the breeding season passes. Resumption of duller plumage after the breeding season is presumably a reflection of the higher mortality suffered by the more brightly colored members of a species. As a further example of conflicts between selection regimes, similar conflicts between individual and group selection are sometimes demanded before the very existence of higher-level selection can be taken as demonstrated.

In final chapters of this book, I will review the arguments for the existence of two parallel but separate hierarchies that appear to arise from the very existence of two sets of distinguishable aspects of organismic phenotypic properties, i.e., the economic and reproductive activities of all organisms. It will be the primary position of this argument that species arise and are maintained through the reproductive activities of organisms. For the moment, however, we will explore further the duality of opinion (sometimes maintained *within* a single school of evolutionary thought) on the very nature of species, seen in light of the fundamental distinction between the two great classes of organismic activity.

Economics and Reproduction: Darwinian and Later Evolutionary Views on the Nature of Species

"Species have a real existence in nature, and a transition from one to another does not exist," or so wrote William Whewell (1837). Whewell was one of the most influential philosophers of his day, and his articulation of the nature of species as viewed by nineteenth-century biologists and philosophers seems fairly representative of pre-Darwinian thinking on the subject. Naturalists had by then been actively engaged in the systematic survey, description, and classification of plants and animals for nearly three quarters of a century (choosing as a starting point the 1758 date of publication of Linnaeus's *Systema*

Naturae). Linnaeus himself thought that species and higher taxa are real.[1] And while in some later publications Linnaeus did concede that there could be connections between species (i.e., that some species could have been derived from others), his basic view remained "Species tot sunt quot diversas formas ab initio produxit Infinitum Ens": "There are as many species as the Creator [Infinite Being] originally fashioned diverse forms." Whewell was merely mouthing tradition when he averred that species are real and share no evolutionary connections.

Darwin's prime task in the *Origin* was to establish the plausibility of the idea that life has had a long history, and that all living things are interconnected in a skein of ancestry and descent ("descent with modification"), as lineages branch and phenotypic innovations are added from time to time in those different branches of the genealogical tree of life. "Descent with modification" is the very antithesis of the second half of Whewell's dictum: "...and a transition from one to another [i.e., species] does not exist." Darwin's idea was precisely the opposite: that a transition between species certainly *does* "exist," i.e., that evolution entails the derivation of descendant species from ancestors.

Yet there remains the issue embodied in the first part of Whewell's statement: "Species have a real existence in nature. . . ." There is no necessary connection between the two statements, for species can "have a real existence" and either give rise to descendant species or not (the latter constitutes the creationist view). Alternatively, species might be construed as artificial, i.e., as *not* real in the sense of being self-organizing, naturally occurring entities, but rather collectivities that exist only in the minds of biologists. If such is the case, then of course it could be true that "transitions from one to another do not exist" (i.e., because species themselves are thought not to exist in any meaningful sense); but it might also be maintained that species *even if they don't really exist as discrete entities* may still be said to give rise to one another. This admittedly rather strange sounding proposition is precisely the view adopted, in the main, by Darwin and, in certain contexts, by the Darwinian tradition in evolutionary biology up to the present time.

Recall that the prime goal in evolutionary biology, from its very beginnings, has been to develop a causal understanding of phenotypic organismic diversity in the biological realm. Natural selection, a mechanism of generation-by-generation change in phenotypic properties, suffices as a first-order solution to the problem of understanding stasis and change in such properties. In this light, it becomes apparent that the phrase "the origin of species" represented (i.e., to Darwin and many of his successors) simply another way of stating the original problem: How do we explain organismic diversity? Mayr (1942) was not the first biologist to remark that Darwin (1859) did not really address the issue of the origin of species in his *On the Origin of Species*. Rather than addressing the issue "How do species become discrete from one another?" Darwin for the most part was concerned to picture evolutionary history as a matter of the smooth and rather progressive transformation of the phenotypic properties of organisms within lineages.

Thus the "origin of species" in Darwinian tradition simply amounts to a matter of accrual of phenotypic change through time. If enough time goes by and enough change accumulates so that later members of a lineage differ from earlier members (as seen, for example, in fossils) to roughly the same extent as members of two closely related, yet separate, modern species might differ, then, according to Darwinian tradition, we can say that a new species has descended from an ancestral one. Were the fossil record complete, with all stages of the transformation faithfully recorded by specimens of intermediate age, we would, as evolutionists, have to be wholly arbitrary in our choice of where we would draw the line—where we would say ancestral species 1 ceased to exist, having been transformed into descendant species 2 (Fig. 4.1).

Yet note that the evolutionary transformation takes place *within lineages,* i.e., within a plexus of reproductively interacting organisms that leaves an unbroken skein of parental ancestry and descent through time. Species are not *wholly* arbitrary because their *lateral boundaries,* so to speak, are clear-cut and reflect an aspect of natural organization. It is just that *through time,* by virtue of the willy-nilly accumulation of phenotypic change, we must chop up the evolving lineage into smaller packages of more or less coherent anatomical organization, calling them "species." And as time continues to go by, even if the lineages do not branch, enough morphological change may accumulate so that we will have to designate new higher taxa—genera, families, and so on.

Thus species seem real enough at any one point in time: especially sympatrically, organisms are usually easily seen as grouped into self-defining reproductive communities, clearly distinct from other reproductive communities. And the organisms within each of these reproductive communities tend to resemble each other more closely than they resemble members of other reproductive communities, no matter how closely they may be related (and especially when comparisons are restricted to members of the same sex and/or age group, which compensates for the effects of sexual dimorphism and the presence of discrete ontogenetic stages in the life histories of organisms). Yet the Darwinian tradition insists that species have no clear-cut temporal di-

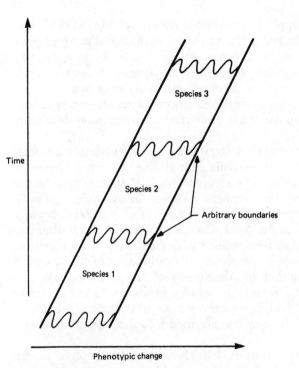

Figure 4.1 Diagram showing a lineage of sexually reproducing organisms divided arbitrarily into time-successive "species" ("chronospecies") on the basis of one or more phenotypic attributes that are undergoing gradual transformation through time.

mension: through time, species are expected as a matter of course to become transformed, to change, to evolve eventually into descendant species in a manner that leaves no possibility for recognizing discrete entities. Thus through time, species are emphemera—and are definitely not to be considered "real." Such continues to be the position of some prominent modern biologists (e.g., Bock, 1979, 1986). Because the concept of time is so deeply and inextricably bound up with the notion of evolution, species, because they are traditionally seen as atemporal, have an extremely ambiguous position within evolutionary biology.

Yet Darwin (1871), in considering contemporaneous species, also maintained that species are "permanent varieties." As we shall see later in this chapter, this was an extremely valuable insight in understanding the context of the occurrence and accumulation of adaptive change in evolutionary history. Thus, in some contexts, Darwin saw species as ephemera, bound to change with the simple passage of time. In other contexts, he saw species as more important, and more stable ("permanent") than "varieties." Indeed, to Darwin, species are *permanent varieties* because they become reproductively isolated from other such varieties. "Varieties" that are not reproductively isolated from one another (i.e., are populations within a single biological species) are far less likely to persist in recognizably intact form than are those "varieties" that have become separate and distinct reproductive communities, i.e., separate species.

Dobzhansky and Mayr: Species and the Modern Synthesis

A few biologists followed the second, muted theme Darwin established, and emphasized the discontinuities evident between closely related, contemporary species. G. J. Romanes, a biologist of the latter half of the nineteenth century, is said to have remarked that "without isolation or the prevention of interbreeding, organic evolution is in no case possible" (quoted, without citation, in Dobzhansky, 1937*a*, p. 228). Romanes and Moritz Wagner, and later systematists such as D. S. Jordan, saw the importance of disjunct geographical distributions, which correlate with the distribution of well-differentiated, yet closely related, pairs or groups of species. Reproductive discontinuities induced by geographical isolation were a minor, but persistent, theme in evolutionary biology (particularly systematics) from the mid-nineteenth century onwards.

But it was not until the modern synthesis was forged starting in the mid-1930s that the theme of discontinuity became thoroughly incorporated into evolutionary biology. Both Dobzhansky (1937*a*, 1941) and later Mayr (1942) stressed that the *twin* themes of evolutionary biology are (1) *diversity* (meaning *phenotypic* diversity, the original problem in evolutionary biology) and (2) *discontinuity* (meaning disruption of the smooth continuum in phenotypic diversity that would be the expected outcome of simple accumulation of adaptive modification through natural selection).

Discontinuity, of course, can arise through simple extinction of intermediates. In a genealogical system in which branching (lineage splitting) occurs along with the ongoing transformation of the components within each lineage, extinction can be expected to terminate many an intermediate branch. But both Dobzhansky and Mayr thought there must be something in addition, something primary, to the gaps they perceived between even the most closely related species living in the present-day faunas and floras of the world. And, precisely because natural selection is expected, by its very nature, to produce a *continuum* of phenotypic diversity, the primary explanation for the *gaps* observed in the distribution of those very same economic adaptations of organisms must, they reasoned, be an outcome of the *repro-ductive* gaps that are also a hallmark of the organization of biotic nature.

And that is the gist of their logic: economic adaptive diversity would be expected to be smoothly continuous. Those gaps in the distribution of economic adaptations not arising from simple extinction of intermediates must therefore arise *causally* as a by-product of the development of reproductive discontinuities, specifically, the development of new reproductive communities from old. Thus both Dobzhansky (1937a) and Mayr (1942) elected to formulate *reproductive* (or *genealogical*) definitions for what species are. Nothing is said (in their definitions) about anatomical similarity; rather, citing the "short" form offered by Mayr (1942, p. 120), species are "groups of actually or potentially interbreeding natural populations, which are reproductively isolated from other such groups." This is the so-called biological species concept.

The biological species concept (BSC) continues to attract severe criticism from a variety of quarters. Thus, sequentially, two schools of modern thought in systematics have questioned the utility of the concept. Pheneticists (e.g., Sokal and Crovello, 1970) have challenged the definition on a variety of operational grounds, essentially alleging that there is nothing inherent in the definition of the BSC that would allow all systematists to identify particular species in practice. And, while it is true that what a species *is* is an issue separate from the methods we might adopt to recognize species (the first being an ontological issue, the second epistemological in nature), nonetheless the BSC, based on reproductive behavior, deviates from the more general use of phenotypic characteristics used to recognize taxa of all other ranks (including, ironically, *subspecies* according to the "new systematics," the methodological companion to the modern synthesis; see Mayr, 1942).

Phylogenetic systematists (cladists) likewise tend to resist the BSC on grounds somewhat similar to those of the pheneticists: in cladistic terms, taxa are defined and recognized strictly in terms of synapomorphies—uniquely shared, phylogenetically derived[2] phenotypic features. These may include reproductive adaptations, but need not be limited to that category of phenotypic properties. In particular, reproductive communality may be maintained in the face of further economic adaptive diversification, such that not all diversified groups within a "species" would be recognized under the BSC. In such instances, some phylogenetic systematists might opt to recognize the smaller, well-differentiated taxa as separate species—despite retention of interbreeding capabilities between such different "species." (see Cracraft, 1988).

A further objection is perhaps even more basic and cuts to the heart of the ontological issue of the nature of species: If species can, in a meaningful way, be said to exist (to have origins, histories, and extinctions)—and especially if we are to conceive biotic nature in such terms that ancestral species give rise to descendant species—then it follows that ancestral species cannot uniquely possess derived characteristics (i.e., of the organismic phenotypes) not shared in the same (or further modified) form with descendants. Thus those species in a sample that are ancestral to other known species cannot be defined and recognized on the basis of (syn)apomorphies, and this violates standard procedure and canons applied to taxa of all other ranks. Ancestors are a problem in cladistics, and even if it is agreed that taxa of rank higher than species do not act as ancestors to other taxa, nonetheless the postulate that species do serve as ancestors to other species raises problems in methodological theory in systematics.[3]

For all the complaints, however, about the difficulty in application of the BSC, evolutionary biologists since the advent of the modern synthesis have tended to accept it as a useful description of nature. As we have seen in the last chapter, however, more recent theoretical discussions of adaptive change through time have tended to overlook the putative existence of discrete, "reproductively isolated" entities (i.e., species) as not particularly germane to the issue of the mode of accumulation of selection-mediated adaptive change, of whatever magnitude, through time. Some biologists (e.g., Levinton, 1988) have even explicitly denied that there is a causal connection between speciation and the accumulation of macroevolutionary adaptive change. And, even within the synthesis, those biologists most concerned with geological time and patterns of transformation of adaptative features— G. G. Simpson most particularly—explicitly rejected the BSC, in part because the BSC as articulated by Dobzhansky and Mayr purposely lacked a temporal dimension (see, e.g., Simpson, as quoted in Mayr, 1980). Simpson also stated (e.g., 1944) that the amount of change typically associated with speciation is so trivial as to be unimportant in the development of theories of large-scale evolutionary change in geological time.

Thus, in many quarters in biology, the nature and existence of species as conceived by some early biologists and culminating in the works of Dobzhansky and Mayr is perceived as either peripheral, irrelevant, or downright contradictory to the methodological formulations and basic concerns of a number of disciplines. These disciplines (as disparate as population genetics and systematics) have one element in common: All focus their primary attention on the phenotypic attributes of organisms—geneticists to get at the hereditary factors ("genes") underlying the phenotypes, systematists to identify and define taxa and to serve as a test of hypotheses of intertaxon interrelatedness. Yet the notion of *discontinuity* as a prime aspect of the organization of biotic nature remains a dominant theme in evolutionary thinking. Morphological gaps, as Dobzhansky and Mayr pointed out, tend (especially among metazoans) to correspond to reproductive gaps. And, though Mayr and Dobzhansky were certainly stalwart neo-Darwinians in their insistence that natural selection produces a smooth continuum in adaptively based phenotypic diversity (and that therefore intermediate forms must always have existed), nonetheless it is the superposition of reproductive isolation (the formation of new, separate reproductive communities from old ones) rather than extinction pure and simple that imposes the discontinuities so obvious even among closely related species.

Mayr (1942) was especially clear that species are "real" entities, remarking that if species were not in some sense real, there would be no reason to develop a theory on how they originate. Yet, Mayr and Dobzhansky (especially evident in Mayr, 1942, p. 153) nonetheless maintained the by then customary Darwinian view of species through time: instead of viewing species strictly as reproductive communities that originate by the budding off of new reproductive communities from old ones (which as an overwhelming rule persist alongside descendants, much as parents persist alongside offspring), Mayr and Dobzhansky were content to see species transforming into descendants by sheer accumulation of transformational change of organismic phenotypic properties through time. It was, in other words, literally true that the BSC was envisioned as holding only for the moment. Through time, a purely *phenotypic resemblance within genealogical lineage* (replete with the reversion to a purely phenetic and arbitrary recognition of where one species ended and its temporal descendant began) was (and continues to be) the ontological conception of choice in the modern synthesis.

"Isolating Mechanisms": Cause and Effect in the Origin of Species

Dobzhansky and Mayr developed the theme, latent in many post-Darwinian writings, that reproductive isolation is a causal forerunner of discontinuity in the distribution of the general adaptive properties of organisms. But such a formulation merely restates the problem, for they then had to consider in detail the cause of *reproductive* discontinuity. The differences between these two evolutionary biologists on the origin of reproductive discontinuity may serve as an introduction to current issues in speciation theory. (A more detailed outline and comparison of Mayr's and Dobzhansky's views on isolating mechanisms can be found in Eldredge, 1985a.)

It was Dobzhansky (1937b) who coined the term "isolating mechanisms." The term was an apt one, for in Dobzhansky's view, there is a critical set of distributional and phenotypic organismic features that act to keep two different species apart, "reproductively isolated" from one another. Both Dobzhansky and Mayr, echoing earlier commentary, saw the importance of geographic isolation. Mayr (and to a significant degree, Dobzhansky in later editions, e.g., 1951) saw geographic isolation as *the* causal first step in producing what he (i.e., Mayr, 1942) referred to as the *bridgeless gaps* (both reproductive and generally morphological) between (especially sympatric) species. Mayr's causal theory is simplicity itself and remains the basic view in modern conceptualizations of speciation: geographic isolation leads to reproductive isolation, which in turn leads to the consolidation and further development of general phenotypic differences between two recently divergent species.

Dobzhansky's view on causality in speciation was critically different from Mayr's in at least one important respect. And though Dobzhansky's rather more complex view never achieved the currency of Mayr's, it sets off all the more starkly the view on species and speciation recently articulated by H. E. H. Paterson (e.g., 1985). For Dobzhansky saw geographic separation and various aspects of organismic phenotypes literally as devices to keep species apart. Rather than as a trigger inducing further anatomical modification, isolating mechanisms in Dobzhansky's mind acted more as a source of consolidation of differences. Dobzhansky (1937a, and in many later publications) imagined species to be perched on "adaptive peaks," occupying niches, and, from the perspective of genetics, maximizing fitness. There is a conflict, from this viewpoint, between optimization of fitness and the accumulation of genetic variation.

Dobzhansky sought to explain reproductive discontinuity in terms of the adaptive value such isolation would bring. He believed the "purpose" of isolation was the avoidance of hybrids with reduced viability, which selection would clearly act against. Thus he saw speciation as a conservative factor, acting against the accumulation of variation, which is, ironically, the raw stuff of further evolution. Dobzhansky's theory was never attractive, because he could not explain the origin of reproductive discontinuity by his "reinforcement" hypothesis (which saw selection acting against hybrids) if there were no overlap in range of two nearly discrete species. Nonetheless, the difference between Mayr's and Dobzhansky's views is important. Dobzhansky saw reproductive isolation arising because it is actually *selected*—because isolation plays a positive role in evolution. Mayr (1942) saw reproductive isolation arising as a side effect (an accidental by-product) of general adaptive and even drift-induced divergence between populations that become, for whatever reason, geographically isolated from one another. For Mayr, reproductive isolation plays no direct evolutionary role and is not selected; yet such isolation has important evolutionary consequences in establishing distinct species. Yet Mayr (1942 and later) saw no difficulty with the term "isolating mechanisms."

Paterson (1985, with references to earlier papers) has done much to clarify the issue of species discontinuity. Rather than pointing to the set of phenotypic features that keep closely related species apart, Paterson (1985) refers to those phenotypic properties of sexually reproducing organisms by which they "recognize" one another as appropriate mates. His analysis does much to clarify previous expositions on "reproductive isolation," and agrees well with both Darwin's earlier discussions of the difference between "natural" and "sexual" selection, and the nature of "secondary sexual characteristics." In other words, Paterson's notion of the *specific mate recognition system* (SMRS) makes the distinction between phenotypic attributes that function economically (i.e., for the maintenance of the organismic soma) and those that are shaped by selection to perform tasks involved in reproduction.[4]

For present purposes, the major significance of Paterson's formulation of the SMRS is that species are conceived as *self-defining (thereby entirely natural) reproductive communities*. Species arise, in Paterson's scheme, in the basic way that Mayr (1942) described, as an outgrowth of geographic isolation. But, unlike Mayr, Paterson sees (sexual) selection *for* mates as the critical element of speciation. Natural selection for economic divergence in isolation may well occur (in Paterson's view), but unless and until the SMRS itself changes in isolation, speciation proper cannot be said to have occurred. As we shall see below, though, Paterson also has argued that when SMRS change occurs, it may well be accompanied by coordinate changes in the economic adaptations of organisms, leading to a punctuated pattern.

Species as Individuals

Yet another, significant component to recent considerations of the very nature of species lies in the suggestion (first made explicit by Ghiselin, 1974; see also Hull, 1976) that species should be considered *individuals*. Ghiselin had in mind a contrast between individuals and *classes*. Individuals are entities with parts; they have names; they are spatiotemporally bounded. They are particularly to be distinguished from unbounded classes. Entities are members of a class strictly by virtue of their possession of some designated feature(s). All atoms of atomic number 79 are designated "gold." Gold is a class, or category, of atomic element that can occur anywhere in the universe and be formed at any time. Each atom of gold, in contrast, is an "individual."

Similarly the taxonomic category (rank) "species" is a class in this sense, while *Homo sapiens,* with its proper name, is an instance of a species; and the species *H. sapiens* is, in this view, an entity—an individual. And though philosophers in general have raised objections to this use of the term "individual," the correlation between Ghiselin's (1974; also Hull, 1976, 1978 for further discussion) class–individual distinction and the fundamental dichotomy in characterization of the basic nature of species as developed earlier in this chapter is obvious. When species are seen as (arbitrarily) delineated clusters of phenotypically similar organisms, they are being treated as classes.[5] Most biologists, convinced that each species is localized in time and space and separated morphologically from other species by gaps, have long since abandoned the extreme position that species are simply classes of similar organisms and artifacts of the classificatory activities of systematists.

A view of species based on cohesion agrees very nicely with Ghiselin's notion that particular species are individuals. Such cohesion is supplied by the reproductive plexus pointed to in the biological species concept and made even more explicit in the work of Paterson, who defines species as the "largest collectivity of organisms with a shared fertilization system" (i.e., shared SMRS). Mayr (1942), when discussing species at a single point in time, referred to them as "real," and very much like *"Paramecium* individuals." Speciation is the beginning—the "birth"—of a new species. Extinction is its termination, its "death." Between birth and death, the properties of organisms that are parts of species may well change, just as individual organisms change between birth and death. Because they have births, histories, and deaths, as well as a source of internal cohesion, species are *spatiotemporally bounded.*

Yet, it remains a contentious point in modern evolutionary theory to refer to species as "individuals." Part of the difficulty is the observational scale on which we perceive species. As parts of a species ourselves,[6] we are very aware of the boundedness of (most) individual organisms, and also of the spaces *between* organisms, which seems to suggest that large-scale entities like species are hardly well-cohered entities. But we must remember that most entities that are taken to be real—most certainly including atoms—likewise consist of space. It is simply much easier to imagine entities on a smaller spatiotemporal scale as "real" than those that exist on relatively large scales. We can see galaxies as individualized entities only when they are so far away as to require telescopic magnification. It was entirely another matter to see the Milky Way as an equivalent individualized entity because, since we are located *within* it, the Milky Way appeared to constitute the entire, rather amorphous, "universe." We biologists may be having an equivalent problem with seeing *Homo sapiens* as a spatio-temporal localized and bounded entity.

Then, too, species, *if they are individuals,* do not appear to be individuals of the same sort that, say, organisms are. Species are rather special kinds of entities, a topic discussed further in Chap. 5. It is essential to understand just what sort of entities species are to specify with any precision the role that they play in nature, including their role in evolution in general, and within macroevolution in particular.

There are further, epistemological points that most likely play at least as strong a role against the general acceptance of the idea that species are "real entities," or "individuals." In particular, neither population geneticists interested in evolutionary theory *nor* systematists concerned with the characterization of taxa and their interrelationships appear to *need* the concept of individuality to carry on with their basic tasks.

Why, then, is it important for evolutionary biologists to take seriously the proposition that species are individuals? The first is empirical: Species seem to be clearly individuated in the fossil record (see below) and, most importantly, appear to be *sorted* in such a way that phylogenetic (evolutionary) patterns appear to be a function of some mechanism of "sorting" as well as a product of natural selection and genetic drift (Chap. 5).

Also, as some biologists (Eldredge and Gould, 1972; Paterson, 1985; Futuyma, 1987) have been discussing, the timing, and degree, of anatomical change in evolution seems very much to be connected to the process of speciation. Thus the phylogenetic transformation of phenotypic properties within species through time, and the disappearance of such features at species extinction, clearly shapes the pattern of phenotypic change through time; but the birth of species appears especially critical in its own right. The notion of "punctuated equilibria" is especially critical in setting the problem out clearly. In conjunction with an understanding of the relationship between variation in economic and reproductive adaptive characteristics of organisms, speciation emerges as a most crucial context of the very process of adaptive change.

Punctuated Equilibria II: Speciation and the Pace of Adaptive Change

In Chap. 3, the discussion of punctuated equilibria was restricted strictly to patterns of transformational change in phylogeny. Now we

must consider the relation between punctuated equilibria and speciation theory—its original explanatory matrix.

As first conceived (Eldredge, 1971; Eldredge and Gould, 1972), the
theory of punctuated equilibria was simply the application of
(allopatric) speciation theory to the pattern of stasis and occasional
brief episodes of phenotypic change that were held to be characteristic
of much of the phylogenetic patterns in the fossil record. Periods of
stasis are attributable primarily to successful habitat tracking by far-
flung species composed of many semi-isolated populations—harking
back to imagery first explored in detail by Wright (1932) and
Dobzhansky, (1937a).

But there is a contentious and almost counterintuitive component to
the suggestion that the fits-and-starts pattern of phylogenetic transformation can be understood as the product of relatively uncommon
speciation events followed by long periods of within-species stability:
the suggestion that most morphological change takes place just prior
to, during, and immediately following the onset of reproductive isolation. On the one hand, if we imagine the stable lineages to represent
species, this is precisely the conclusion we must come to. On the other
hand, there are severe methodological problems of species recognition
in the fossil record, including a problem in circularity pertaining to
precisely the issue of coordinate timing of speciation and morphological transformation. And, finally, there is the most interesting question of all: Why should economic adaptive change be correlated with
the origin of a descendant reproductive community from an ancestral
reproductive community?

Let us consider first the formidable epistemological problem of species recognition in the fossil record. Recall that perhaps the prepon-
derance of post-Darwinian history has seen species as collections of
anatomically similar organisms, such that species are arbitrarily delineated segments of continuously evolving lineages, in which the
morphological features of component organisms are undergoing continual modification through time. In such a conceptualization of species and the evolutionary process, transformation of morphology is the
direct, unambiguous "cause" of speciation. In this light, species recognition is difficult in paleontology only because transformation blurs
the distinction between species, whereas the gaps between two closely
related species are far more readily perceived at any one time and
place.

But suppose we adopt some form of the BSC concept, i.e., see species
as reproductive communities. In such a case, we might rely on whatever morphological features that separate species consistently, regardless of the adaptive nature (i.e., the function) of the features, so
long, that is, as the gaps in morphology correspond to the actual

bounds of the reproductive community. Morphology is a guide here, while reproductive isolation, established initially through geographic isolation, is the "cause" of speciation.

In the fossil record, it is obviously quite difficult to specify with assurance what the different "reproductive communities" at any one time and place are, let alone to trace such reproductive communities (i.e., species) through time with confidence. Yet the situation is not as hopeless as sometimes suggested (e.g., Levinton and Simon, 1980). Modern organisms (for example, mollusks cast up along the strandline at high tide) can in most cases readily be sorted into morphologically well demarcated clusters. There is little difficulty in demonstrating that these clusters correspond exactly with functioning reproductive communities—local demes belonging to discrete species—just offshore, below the waves. Invertebrate paleontologists can make a similar collection of easily sorted, morphologically discrete mollusks, brachiopods, trilobites, etc., on any given Paleozoic bedding plane. We can assume that, were the information available, the same overwhelming correspondence between morphological clusters and discrete breeding communities would emerge as is readily seen in modern examples.

There are two sources of error here: there is the danger both of overestimating and of underestimating the true number of species in a sample, inferring, that is, the number of reproductive communities by assuming that the number of morphologically distinguishable sets of organisms corresponds exactly with the number of discrete reproductive communities present. Sibling species (morphologically very similar, closely related species) will be overlooked; and polymorphisms will lead to an *over*estimation of the true number of species present in any sample. Nonetheless, experience with sympatric demes of species collected in a local habitat (where most of the species are not particularly closely related, as the overwhelming rule) shows a strong correlation between numbers of morphologically delineated clusters of organisms, on the one hand, and number of reproductive communities present, on the other. The same may be assumed for any contemporaneous collection in the fossil record.

Stasis—the persistence of morphological complexes with little significant (lasting, or directionally accumulating) variation—conveniently allows such morphological "packages" recognized at any one moment to be recognized for considerable lengths of geological time. Species remain recognizably "the same" (i.e., in terms of the phenotypic properties of component organisms), in many instances for millions of years. Note that stasis is not a prerequisite for conceptualizing species as individuals; but stasis does reinforce the idea that species are spatiotemporally bounded entities, simply because it is, as a rule, so easy to identify a species through more than a single time plane. In other words, based on the work of paleontologists (cited in the preceding chapter) on stasis, the Darwinian expectation that species will invariably and inevitably continue to undergo morphological transformation is not confirmed. Far from transforming themselves out of existence as a matter of course, species tend to exhibit great morphological conservatism.

But what does such overall stasis imply for the view of species as reproductive communities? Can we not imagine that behavioral and physiological change might accumulate even in the absence of pronounced anatomical change? If so, interbreeding might well not have been possible were end members of a long-lived species (separated, say, by millions of years) hypothetically to be brought together. Yet, in such an imaginary experiment, what counts is the ongoing skein of reproductive interaction through time. The SMRS may indeed change through time, but there is lineage continuity throughout. A new species begins when a new community is severed off from an ancestral reproductive community. It persists until all member organisms are dead.

Yet, recognizing species, *defined* as reproductive communities, strictly through the economic attributes of organisms remains somewhat unsatisfactory. That is why rare situations in the fossil record, in which elements of the SMRS are preserved, are so important. Such instances demonstrate that, *in principle,* species truly can be recognized in the fossil record, utilizing the same criteria of recognition used by the organisms themselves. An example is provided by Vrba (1980, 1984b; see Chap. 5 for discussion), whose analysis of antelope phylogenetic patterns is partially based on horn morphology and its status as part of antelope specific mate-recognition systems.

A Classification of Speciation Models

Before addressing a fundamental problem right at the interface of micro- and macroevolution (viz., Why should morphological change in general be concentrated at speciation events?), we must first summarize the foregoing in terms of causal processes in speciation. The resulting classification of types of speciation will be considerably different from other recent classifications, which we shall also briefly review. The point of such a classification is to reveal the basic causal structure of adaptive change in general, leading to a consideration of the interactions between economic and genealogical (reproductive) adaptive change that lie at the heart of speciation and its relation to morphological change in evolution.

We have seen that there are two basic conceptualizations of the overall nature of species that are both consistent with, and fundamental aspects of, the Darwinian heritage of evolutionary biology. Species can be seen, first and foremost, as collections of phenotypically similar organisms, albeit also as members of reproductively coherent lineages. Or, we may emphasize (as Dobzhansky and Mayr were the first to do unequivocally) the reproductive community nature of species—but not losing sight of the fact that, in spite of great variation within some species, organisms within a species (especially those of the same sex and age class) resemble each other more closely than they resemble members of the same sex and age class of other species. Thus there is a general relation between reproductively coherent communities and phenotypically similar clusters of organisms. In general, one set of features may be used to estimate the other. Phenotypic resemblance is used more commonly than SMRS features to determine species identities, simply because SMRS data are more difficult to gather, even with Recent organisms. But species identification is an epistemological matter. Ontologically, what we think species *are*, fundamentally, naturally colors how we think they originate. And we should note that, in general, the distinction between "overall phenotypic similarity" and "SMRS" corresponds, respectively, very closely to the distinction between the economic and reproductive adaptations of organisms.

Ever since Mayr's (1942) discussion of speciation, evolutionary biologists have focused their classification of "modes" of speciation around the primary means of establishment of reproductive isolation. The primary dichotomy, as perceived by Mayr and maintained to the present time, is between *allopatric* and *sympatric* speciation. The contrast is between reproductive isolation arising from an initial causal impetus of simple geographic isolation (allopatric, or geographic, speciation) and reproductive disjunction arising in the face of regular contact among organisms (sympatric, or *nongeographic,* speciation).

While Mayr (1942, and many later references) steadfastly denied the possibility of true sympatric speciation, later authors included reference at least to its possible occurrence in their classifications. Thus, in a widely used scheme, Bush (1975) contrasted allopatric speciation (with two subtypes) with sympatric and "parapatric"[7] modes. The origin of reproductive barriers between organisms that do have regular contact necessitates spontaneous appearance of phenotypic (including behavioral and physiological, as well as simple morphological) differences that impede reproduction among two subsets of an ancestral species. For example, the most commonly cited such spontaneous inhibitor of successful reproduction—at least in parapatric models (White's [1968] "stasipatric" speciation)—is chromosomal rearrangement.

In an interesting departure from the geographically based type of categorization of speciation modes, Templeton (1981) contrasted what he termed the "divergence" from "transilience" modes. Templeton (1981, p. 26) noted that geographically based classifications of speciation tend to lump some diverse population genetics processes, while artificially dividing others. The point of departure of Templeton's classification, accordingly, was the processes of population genetics. According to Templeton (1981, p. 27), the "divergence" category includes instances in which "isolating barriers evolve in a continuous (but not necessarily slow) fashion, with some form of natural selection, either directly or indirectly, being the driving force leading to reproductive isolation. Transilient modes involve a discontinuity in which some sort of selective barrier is overcome by other evolutionary forces. In a somewhat oversimplified sense, divergence occurs because of selection, transilience in spite of selection."

Templeton's "divergence" modes include the initiation of reproductive isolation by an extrinsic barrier (normally, geographic isolation); he includes "clinal" and "habitat" as submodes, as well. Under "transilience," Templeton lists "genetic" (i.e., rapid shifts between stable states of genetic systems arising from founder effects), chromosomal events, and the formation of new species through hybridization between "incompatible parental species" (two distinct submodes).

Yet it would appear that yet another scheme is called for, one that embraces as its first dichotomy the recognition of distinctly different fundamental conceptualizations of what species *are*. The postsynthesis classifications all emphasize (understandably and correctly) the various ways that reproductive isolation is attained. Reproductive isolation is the sine qua non of speciation in all these schemes. However, the view that species are, in a temporal sense, simply arbitrarily recognized subdivisions of evolving continua is clearly present in all writings of the synthesis (Mayr, 1942, p. 15; Simpson, 1944, 1953, virtually throughout). It remains a dominant conceptualization of species in contemporary evolutionary biology, especially, though not exclusively, in the paleontological literature (e.g., Gingerich, 1976; but see also Dawkins, 1986, p. 264).

Moreover, *how* reproductive discontinuity arises might more reasonably be classified according to *what subset of organismal phenotypic properties* are primarily involved; this entails a recognition of different causal relations between economic and reproductive (genealogical) sets of organismic phenotypic (and underlying genotypic) properties. Whether the modifications arise through drift in spite of selection or directly through selection seems of less significance than the basic nature of the changes themselves.

Thus a natural classification of "speciation" suggests itself (Table

4.1). We need, first, to distinguish the two categories of species still current in evolutionary biology: (1) species as products of the spatiotemporal transformation of phenotypic and underlying genotypic properties (so that new species are simply subdivisions of a continuum designated by systematists or paleontologists) and (2) species that are seen as reproductive communities (so that speciation is an actual process in nature and entails the disjunction between ancestral and descendant reproductive communities).

Within the latter category, there are two fundamentally distinct modes of the origin of reproductive discontinuity. The first is basically the "standard" model, replete (as briefly reviewed above) with many subtypes. The model in all its forms, however, sees the origin of reproductive discontinuity as arising from transformation of some aspect(s) of the general economic (somatic) systems of organisms. In its simplest form, what is intended is that enough genetically based economic change accrues that reproduction would be impossible. If enough adaptive change occurs, in other words, there is sufficient genetic incompatibility to prevent successful mating. A recent review of speciation mechanisms (Barton and Charlesworth, 1984), for example, is wholly given over to this view. In all versions of this "standard" model, speciation develops as an outgrowth of such differentiation, though Templeton's distinction between divergence and transilience is useful here, with its recognition that transilience occurs in spite of the continuum of adaptive divergence, superposing genetic discontinuities in the face of continuity.

TABLE 4.1   A Classification of Speciation Modes Based on Species Ontology and Causal Relations of Economic and Genealogical Phenotypic (and Underlying Genotypic) Properties of Organisms

I. Species as arbitrary subsets of evolving continua	Speciation is a matter of human recognition of artificial subdivisions of a continuum of phenotypic adaptive differentiation through time.
II. Species as reproductive communities	Speciation is the establishment of reproductive isolation.
A. Transformation of *economic* phenotypic (and underlying genotypic) attributes	Speciation occurs through accumulation of sufficient change to prevent reproduction (various models, including temporal and geographical divergence, with or without extrinsic barriers; via drift and/or selection).
B. Transformation of SMRS	Speciation occurs through drift and/or selection-mediated change in SMRS.
C. Combination model	Economic transformation is partially incorporated into SMRS (see text).

Yet Templeton's distinction between divergence and transilience also applies to the other great subdivision of the reproductive discontinuity category of the present classification. In this division, we take Paterson's (1985) characterization of the SMRS as the essential ingredient of what a species *is*. It follows that speciation is, at base, a matter of fragmentation of the SMRS. Such can surely occur in a variety of ways, including some that would be called "divergence," and others "transilience" in Templeton's classificatory scheme. Here, the causal pathways leading to reproductive discontinuity are drastically different from the *economic divergence leads to reproductive divergence* scheme of the "standard" outlook: in Paterson's scheme, the SMRS and the rest of the (economic) phenotype may be expected to vary independently (though in point of fact they usually do not). In any case, SMRS discontinuity is a result of selection (or even drift) at work *directly on the SMRS* and is *not* a function of economic divergence. Recognizing that it is the SMRS itself that is minimally required to be modified for speciation to occur has the important additional consequence that we can investigate *both* the implications of *economic* change for *SMRS* change and the implications, as yet little explored but potentially of great importance to unraveling the very context of (macro)evolutionary adaptive change, of *SMRS* change for the development of *economic* adaptive change.

There is one final subcategory of speciation mechanisms. Recalling Darwin's (1871) original discussion of secondary sexual characters, we can see that economic change may lead directly to SMRS change *if* such economic change is co-opted as part of the SMRS; if, in other words, prospective mates learn to recognize one another because of, or even in spite of, changes in outward appearance occasioned by adaptive transformation of some aspect of the phenotype (a situation pertinent especially to Metazoa), the distinction between the two basic subtypes of "true" speciation is to some extent blurred.

It is obvious that there is a direct relation between the idea that speciation is nothing more than the accumulation of adaptive divergence and the view that reproductive isolation arises as a consequence of such divergence. It is true, as set forth above, that Dobzhansky and Mayr stipulated that species are, at base, reproductive communities. They came to this conclusion because, although natural selection generates continua of adaptive diversity, nature appears to be divided into more or less discrete "packages" of anatomical diversity. Reproductive discontinuity, they concluded, must be causally prior to adaptive discontinuity. Yet reproductive discontinuity is achieved by simple divergence—the accumulation of adaptive (phenotypic) differences in the genotype—through the imposition (in both Dobzhansky's and Mayr's views) of geographic isolation. The prime motor of evolution-

ary change remains selection (and to some extent drift), and discontinuity arises only when reproductive systems are accidentally disrupted. Dobzhansky went further, claiming that there is an economic
adaptive "purpose" to reproductive discontinuity. Regardless of which
particular subset of views is admitted, however, and regardless of the
Mayr-Dobzhansky definition of species as reproductive communities,
speciation (just as in the original phyletic transformation model) remains primarily the side effect of (adaptive, in the main) economic evolutionary change.

Paterson's views on the SMRS raise the possibility that the vecto-
rial arrows of causality may be more complex: that changes specifically in the reproductive phenotypes of organisms, and the appearance
in this manner of new species, may be causally antecedent to the development and/or conservation of economic adaptive change. It is to
these possibilities that we now turn, to conclude this chapter on
speciation and evolutionary change.

Speciation and Adaptive Change:
Interactions Between Genealogical and
Economic Components of Organismal
Phenotypes

Analysis of the relation between speciation and adaptive change in
general centers on the interrelations between economic and reproductive aspects of the phenotype. As a "null hypothesis," we might expect
a considerable degree of independence in evolutionary transformation
between the two sets of characteristics. Indeed, that reproductive and
economic components of the phenotype are largely independent in
their rates of phylogenetic transformation is the very basis of the
usual categorization of heterochronic modes (Chap. 6). In the context
of adaptive transformation and speciation, Vrba (1980) presented a
useful 2 by 2 contingency table (Fig. 4.2) that sets forth the possible
relations between degree (or rate) of morphological change, on the one
hand, and the attainment of "reproductive isolation" on the other. Little or no (economic) adaptive change may be apparent between two
closely related but reproductively distinct species; conversely, there
may be a great deal of (adaptively based) phenotypic diversity within
a single, widespread reproductive community—a single species.

But closer analysis quickly reveals that the four quadrants of Vrba's
contingency diagram are by no means occupied uniformly. There is no
equal probability for each square to be occupied, as our initial null hypothesis would lead us to expect. Rather, and as we have already reviewed at length, adaptive transformation of economic (non-SMRS)
aspects of the phenotype seems very definitely to be associated to a

	Speciation	
	Within species	Between species

Morphology	Discernible differentiation absent	A	B
	Discernible differentiation present	C	D

Figure 4.2 Vrba's diagram depicting the "relationship between morphological differentiation and speciation." (Redrawn from Vrba, 1980, Fig. 5, p. 68)

significant degree with speciation events. Recall that there is a strong tradition in evolutionary biology simply to note such change and then conclude that new species have appeared in a rather abrupt manner; this is the view that species are simply designated collections of phenotypically similar organisms—the outcomes of a general process of adaptive change. We are considering here, in contrast, the proposition that SMRS and general (economic) adaptive change are quasi-independent, yet to some extent interrelated. The task now is to specify the causal nature of the correlation between the two.

How can the 2 by 2 contingency table that stresses the independence of SMRS and economic adaptive change be reconciled with the empirical results indicating that economic *and* genealogical (SMRS) adaptive change in fact seem to go hand in hand in evolution? There are several possibilities, all of which involve causal relations between economic and reproductive adaptive change. As we have seen, the "standard" view is that reproductive isolation arises strictly as an accidental outgrowth of the accumulation of economic adaptive change. Altokhov (1982, p. 1168) perhaps summarized this line of thought most succinctly when he wrote: "Reproductive isolation, an important criterion of species, is viewed in this model (i.e. standard synthesis model) as only a by-product of such differentiation." The causal pathways involved are (1) morphological differentiation, followed by (2) geographic isolation, leading to (3) reproductive isolation, which further leads to (4) discernible gaps in morphological variation among closely related species. Economic adaptive differentiation remains the initial mover; reproductive isolation—i.e., adaptive differences in the SMRS—has the secondary effect of making the economic differences more pronounced.

But should the principle of independent variation in economic and SMRS phenotypic features lead necessarily to an equal distribution of probabilities in the 2 by 2 contingency table? Is there any reason, in other words, to predict a systematic departure from such expectation? Might we expect to find (as nature itself seems to suggest we *do* find; see Chap. 3) that (1) little or no accumulation of economic change occurs in the absence of SMRS change, but that (2) in the presence of SMRS change, no, little, moderate, and even large amounts of economic change are present? Put another way, is SMRS change necessary (but not sufficient) for the occurrence and accrual of substantial economic adaptive change? Is there any reason to suppose that SMRS change actually leads to adaptive economic change?

There are two general categories of causal effect that SMRS change might have that may be expected to foster economic adaptive change: (1) conservation of existing variation and (2) the triggering of additional adaptive modification. The first of these possibilities has been discussed, off and on, ever since Darwin (1871) pointed out that species are, in effect, "permanent varieties."

Speciation and the Conservation of Economic Adaptive Change

Dobzhansky (1937a and later) has been the most prominent proponent of the view that species and speciation figure importantly in the conservation of adaptive change, as when he insists that reproductive isolation between species helps keep each species perched more precisely on its adaptive peak. The effect is to prevent formation of "inharmonious gene combinations" (i.e., between species), though the further effect would be to reduce further possibilities of evolutionary change by limiting the number of possible gene combinations. Among more recent writers, Futuyma (1987) and Vrba (1985, 1988) have also argued that variation within species tends to be ephemeral; only when there is reproductive isolation—or SMRS change according to Vrba (1988) in agreement with Paterson (e.g., 1985)—can phenotypic variation be said to have become truly *phylogenetic,* i.e., added to the evolutionary history of a taxon, with prospects of further transmission and transformation in later descendants.

Dobzhansky (1937a) based much of his description of nature, and hence much of his evolutionary theory, on the work of Sewall Wright (see Eldredge, 1985a, Chap. 2 for full discussion). Wright, though primarily a theoretician and mathematical analyst of experimental results, depicted biological nature in a manner that has seemed strikingly apt and accurate to a number of later biologists. Wright (e.g., 1931, 1932; see also 1982, 1988) saw species for the most part to be divided up into many quasi-isolated local "colonies"—later to be called *demes*. Demes are local breeding communities within species. It is supposed that there is some gene flow between the demes. Demes, further, are themselves notoriously ephemeral: they become extinct and reform with great frequency, reflecting local biotic and physical environmental conditions.

It is within demes, integrated as local populations (*avatars:* Damuth, 1985) within local ecosystems, that natural selection is maintaining, or modifying, the economic attributes of organisms. In such a context, for example, polymorphic, geographically variable species develop, i.e., through the adaptive divergence of local populations within a species spread out over a considerable geographical area. It is in such a context, moreover, that the Red Queen model of Van Valen (1973) pertains, even though the model as originally developed imagined gradual change throughout an entire species. Instead, the picture Van Valen developed is applicable to local ecosystems; the adaptive effect on any given focal deme remains local: i.e., there will be no effect (as a rule, in any case) on the adaptive modifications within other demes of the same species, which are undergoing their own, slightly different adaptive histories in other ecological systems. Stasis (the specieswide tendency *not* to exhibit concerted, and especially directional, change) is partly a matter of continued "habitat recognition" in the face of environmental change (and shifting locale of habitats), as previously discussed. In the present context, deriving from Wright's picture of biotic nature, it is also apparent that no concerted net directional change as a rule accrues within a species because local demes are each undergoing slightly different (possibly parallel, but equally possibly divergent) (economic) adaptive histories. And demes, moreover, are themselves ephemeral. Hence Darwin's observation, echoed sporadically by evolutionists ever since, that varieties are ephemeral and species rather more "permanent."

Thus genealogical change is necessary to inject economic adaptive change into the phylogenetic stream. Without SMRS change, much economic change is simply lost. This in itself is an important element to the general context of the generation of adaptive change, an element missing from discussions of adaptation that ignore the organization of nature into species.

Why is there a spectrum in degree of economic differentiation associated with SMRS change? Why, in other words, are there entire clades of relatively morphologically uniform species while there is great divergence in others? Following the argument above, it could be supposed that SMRS change merely conserves what variation has been generated within a single (ancestral) species, whether it is a lot (in a polymorphic species) or relatively little (as in sibling species). Yet there seem to be additional elements in the *conservation of variation* side of the causal role played by SMRS change in economic adaptive change.

Even within a single species, the interplay between SMRS and economic adaptive change can apparently begin the process of SMRS-caused accumulation of economic adaptive differentiation. For example, Ryan and Wilczynski (1988) have convincingly demonstrated variation in aspects of the SMRS (mating calls and receptors) between neighboring populations of the cricket frog *Acris crepitans* in Texas. Demonstrating assortative mating in conjunction with this variation, they have discussed the implications such variation would have on the accumulation of general "genetic differentiation" among these populations.

Another line of thought is suggested by Lewis's (1966) work, in which he painted a rather graphic picture of speciation in flowering plants. Contrasting two models of speciation (one involving the by now familiar one of gradual adaptive divergence, the other a model of rapid chromosomal differentiation leading to hybrid sterility), Lewis (1966) argued that, under the latter model, resultant small populations would be "genetically impoverished." But, with their full reproductive isolation, there would be opportunity for "reworking" of their genetic systems.

Lewis's (1966) discussion centers around sudden disruption of mate recognition systems. Lewis believes that though they are unlikely events, relatively sudden disruptions (particularly in chromosomal arrangements) are actually more likely than gradual divergence in flowering plants. The picture he paints, then, is one that contrasts reproductive with economic divergence. Critically, as Lewis (1966, p. 169) points out, there is little ecologically (in general, phenotypically) to distinguish parental species from small populations of reproductively isolated organisms that arise in such a fashion. Thus his discussion raises the issue of *survival* of newly reproductively isolated populations. What may well be at stake is not so much the difficulty of forming "reproductively isolated" populations (i.e., disrupting SMRSs) as their subsequent survival and long-term participation as members of a genealogical clade.

Lewis himself implies that the probability of survival of small populations increases with greater ecological differentiation of the small, descendant new species from the parental species. With little to differentiate a new species from its more populous and ecologically identical parent, there is little chance the restricted descendant will gain a foothold and survive. It is simply an ecological "clone" of the already well established parental species.

Thus, if it is true that newly isolated species have a greater probability of survival the greater their *economic* differences with the parental species, the phylogenetic record will be biased automatically towards an accumulation of more well differentiated, rather than less well differentiated, species. It is they who tend to survive. Mere disruption of SMRS, with little else to foster survival, is insufficient over the long run for the accumulation of new species.

The *conservation* of economic change through SMRS disruption is clearly of great importance in the accumulation of adaptive change in phylogeny. Yet, insofar as such conservation is concerned, it makes little formal difference *how* reproductive isolation is achieved. Though Lewis's (1966) distinction between economic change and purely reproductive transformation highlights the interaction between the two classes of organismic attributes, in any case it remains the function of "reproductive isolation" to capture whatever economic differentiation has already occurred. It is another matter altogether to assert that SMRS disruption is a *cause* of, or at least fosters, actual *further economic transformation*, i.e., rather than simply the conservation of transformation that has already occurred. Yet such remains a distinct possibility.

Speciation and the Generation of Economic Adaptive Change

Paterson (1985, and earlier references cited therein) and Vrba (e.g., 1985, 1988) have argued that the model of speciation *via* SMRS disruption implies a "punctuated" pattern of phylogenetic change in general. The reason seems to be that it is spatial isolation, reflecting environmental change, that leads to SMRS disruption and, simultaneously and coincidentally, to economic change. SMRS change reflects the same sort of abrupt response to environmental change that may also be represented by economic adaptive change.

Other authors have gone further, suggesting that SMRS disruption actually may *induce* economic adaptive change, i.e., rather than merely occur in concert with it, or lead to the conservation of economic adaptive change. For example, following the lead of Mayr (1942, and many later publications), Eldredge and Gould (1972; 1974 and thereafter) have argued that small populations near the periphery of the range of an ancestral population may be ideally suited to rapid adaptive change following the onset of reproductive isolation. Particularly because peripheral populations are (assumed to be) at the extremes of ecological tolerance for members of the parental species, such adaptive differences already developed may well be expected to become accentuated, given only the requisite genetic potential: selection may well be expected to adjust rapidly the newly isolated and rather small population (small at least when compared with the parental species as a whole) to the edaphic conditions at the periphery of the parental species's range. Thus SMRS disruption under such conditions may readily be imagined to act as a "release," or a "trigger" to further adaptive change the better to fit the particular ecological conditions at the periphery of the parental species's range.

Mayr's model of peripatric speciation (i.e., of allopatric speciation accomplished by small-sized populations at the periphery of the ancestral species's range) is particularly compelling because the problems of accumulation of adaptive (i.e., economic) change in species consisting of many semi-isolated demes are obviated. In such a situation, the deme and local ecological population are roughly one and the same. It is when a new, fledgling species is still small and not yet organized in the manner of a well-established and broadly distributed species that adaptive change might be expected to be rapid and, because the species is already reproductively isolated from the parental species, conserved.

Bock (1970, 1972, 1979) has argued that interaction between parent and daughter species *after* "reproductive isolation" has been attained, and when the two first become sympatric (*neosympatry*), is the source of significant selection forces leading to adaptive change. His point bears resemblance to Dobzhansky's (1937a) arguments on reinforcement, which, however, see such interaction as necessary for selection to *lead* to reproductive isolation. Bock sees such selection as restricted to the post-full-isolation phase. Nonetheless, both biologists cite such competitive interaction as a direct impetus of adaptive change connected with the speciation process.

The conclusion seems inescapable: significant adaptive change in sexually reproducing lineages accumulates only in conjunction with occasional disruptions of the SMRSs. Even were it imagined that long-term, gradual accumulation of economic change in itself would lead to SMRS disruption, such a process seems far too slow to account for the observed patterns of adaptive change that are empirically documented, and reviewed in Chap. 3. It is the independent disruption of the SMRS that underlies the conservation of preexisting evolutionary variation and also serves as the inducement for the generation of additional adaptive economic transformation.

Other authors have developed related models, arguing that speciation must involve, or even literally be an underlying *cause* of, significant amounts of phenotypic, and underlying genotypic, change. The point of the present discussion is that there is an entire spectrum from slight to marked economic phenotypic change in conjunction with SMRS disruption. The economic change may be induced by the SMRS change; or the two may reflect a simultaneous, but independent, response to isolation and environmental change; or economic change may simply be conserved by SMRS disruption (where otherwise it may have been doomed to disappear as ephemeral within-species variation). There is no necessary implication, in the present discussion, that speciation *necessarily* entails marked amounts of economic morphological change; but the converse is held to be true: *marked economic change is unlikely to appear phylogenetically unless accompanied by SMRS disruption.*

The present discussion, then, is based on the fact that the economic phenotypic differences between closely related species are usually not prodigious. (If there is a latent gradualism in macroevolution, it is in the stepwise accumulation *among species* of rather slight phenotypic differences.) Nonetheless, to close the present discussion, it is to be noted that many authors have explicitly developed models to account for large-scale phenotypic changes associated with speciation. Goldschmidt (1940), for example, developed his notions of saltatory evolution because patterns of variation *among* closely related species involved phenotypic attributes other than those observed to be varying *within* those species (of the gypsy moth genus *Lymantria*). Carson (e.g., 1982) developed a model of cascading speciation which likewise cited the impetus of genetic isolation to considerable adaptive economic change—relatively rapidly (though certainly not in a saltatory mode). Lewis (1966) states that new species arising suddenly may occasionally accumulate sufficient novelty to lead to significant departures in the morphological evolution of a clade. And Stanley (1979), in speaking of *quantum speciation,* directly addresses the possibility that rather large adaptive differences may appear in the context of a single speciation event. The point here is neither to endorse nor to reject any of these specific models, but simply to acknowledge their existence, and to acknowledge, as well, the reality that significant morphological change *can* accompany speciation. But the "punctuational" view is not based on a claim that large-scale change *must* accompany speciation. Indeed, most speciation events entail rather modest amounts of change. But it *is* apparent that large-scale change among metazoans and metaphytes is highly unlikely in the absence of speciation, defined as the independent disruption of SMRSs.[8]

Notes to Chapter 4

1. Specifically, Linnaeus thought that the *taxon gives the characters,* rather than the *characters give the taxon*—indication that he felt that taxa are real and that what we

now call the phenotypic properties of organisms stand simply as handy means of recognizing and defining the taxa. Viewed the other way around, i.e., if we adopt the position that the *characters give the taxon*, there is a strong tendency to view taxa merely as assemblages of similar organisms, perhaps even arbitrarily designated by the whims of the particular systematist who happens to be studying a given group. To this date, many biologists persist in the belief that species are simply arbitrarily delineated clusters of similar organisms, i.e., having no particular "reality" and being defined solely on shared possession of certain phenotypic properties.

2. Hennig (1966) is the generally accepted source for the formulation of the basic principles of what he termed *phylogenetic systematics*, later dubbed *cladistics*. Some later cladists explicitly eschew a phylogenetic context for their work and are variously termed "transformed" or "pattern" cladists. Be that as it may, no cladist of whatever stripe known to me denies that "shared derived features" are anything but evolutionary (i.e., phylogenetic) novelties shared by the ancestral and later members of a particular lineage.

3. Species—and higher taxa—when viewed as discrete entities do have properties unique to themselves as individuals: their geographical and temporal distributions. That systematists traditionally utilize the properties of *organisms* to define and recognize *taxa*, however, contributes heavily to the supposition that taxa of all ranks are merely collections of organisms and do not constitute spatiotemporally bounded entities in their own right. For more on species and higher taxa as "individuals," see below.

4. As Darwin (1871) himself noted, "secondary sexual characteristics" frequently represent a complex commingling of reproductive and nonreproductive aspects of the phenotype. General aspects of the soma may take on added roles in sexual behavior. Paterson's SMRS consists of all phenotypic attributes actually used by mates to "recognize" an appropriate mate. These may be any aspect of morphology or behavior; moreover, "recognition" obviously need not imply cognition or even deliberate "choice." Gametes of all sexually reproducing organisms "recognize" one another chemically, and in the case of many sessile invertebrates, chemical recognition among gametes may constitute most of the SMRS of a species.

5. Some cladists have even suggested that, in principle, were organisms sharing the properties of species on earth to be found elsewhere in the universe, they would have to be considered the same species. This makes any *particular* species equivalent to a class, like *gold*.

6. Actually, demes are parts of species; organisms are parts of demes.

7. "Parapatric" refers to populations or species distributed allopatrically but with broad zones of contact.

8. Dobzhansky (1937a, 1941) ended the first two editions of *Genetics and the Origin of Species* with a discussion of asexual "species," necessary, in his view, because he had argued so strenuously that the adaptive importance of "reproductive" isolation is to keep species perched on their own separate "adaptive peaks." How, then, could asexual organisms also have obvious phenotypic gaps separating them? The answer, in retrospect, seems clear: Evolution in truly asexual organisms involves separate clonal lineages *which are only distinguishable when a mutationally based viable novelty actually appears*. The gaps are mutationally based, and the hordes of separate clonal lineages are simply ignored unless and until such a novelty appears. In like fashion, monophyletic taxa are only defined and recognized when marked by an evolutionary novelty—a synapomorphy—that allows a systematist to "see" them. Otherwise, the lineages arising out of distinct species not so distinctly marked remain subsumed under unsatisfactory higher-taxon names (the familiar problem of plesiomorphic stem taxa) which range in size from genera—e.g., *Hyracotherium*, the classic stem horse genus (MacFadden, 1976)—to kingdoms (e.g., Prokaryota).

Yet a similar problem with asexual organisms would appear to affect the argument of the importance of SMRS disruption for the accumulation of adaptive change in evolution in general. There is, after all, no coordinate SMRS change in non-sexually reproducing organisms. True asexuality is rare, yet it is known, and adaptive change does mark the history of such "clone clades" just as it does lineages of sexually reproducing organisms. Yet the answer to Dobzhansky's difficulty is also the answer to this objection arising from asexual species: we only see clonal lineages that are stamped by viable change, and such must be mutationally based. Thus, even though prokaryotes over the last 3.5 billion years are marked by substantial differences in basic metabolic pathways (more than likely developed early in their phylogenetic history)—so that we cannot say that "macroevolution" does not occur among such simple organisms—the differences between the major lineages must have accumulated through single mutational steps. Viable changes, if conserved, lead to the establishment of vast plexuses of clones.

5

Species
and
Macroevolution

G. G. Simpson (e.g., 1944) frequently characterized the amount of phenotypic change associated with speciation as "trivial." Simpson viewed species simply as the smallest conveniently recognizable increment of change within a lineage. Yet even biologists who view speciation as the attainment of "reproductive isolation"—whether through simple economic adaptive divergence in allopatry or through SMRS adaptive modification—agree in general that the amount of economic adaptive differences between two closely related species is usually not great. Closely related species seldom differ to the degree generally associated with "macroevolution."

The last chapter concluded with the proposition that the relation between economic and genealogical (SMRS) adaptive change is not symmetrical in the evolutionary process. Specifically, among sexual organisms, little economic adaptive change accrues within lineages in the absence of divergence in SMRS (i.e., the splitting of reproductive lineages). SMRS divergence, on the other hand, is accompanied by a spectrum of degrees of economic adaptive change, ranging from little or none (sibling species) to moderate amounts (i.e., the relatively small differences usually observed between closely related species) to less common instances in which economic change associated with speciation is marked.

Thus the relation between speciation and macroevolutionary economic adaptive change focuses on two parameters: rate of speciation within a lineage and amount of change associated with speciation events. Much speciation with modest amounts of accompanying change may lead to the accumulation of as much economic adaptive change as fewer events accompanied by relatively greater amounts of divergence per speciation event (Fig. 5.1). But the resultant phylogenetic patterns created by these two possibilities differ in obvious and predictable ways.

Saltationists—such as the geneticist Richard Goldschmidt and the paleontologist Otto Schindewolf—spoke of relatively rare events in which large-scale genetically based phenotypic change occurs virtually as a single (genetic) event. In contrast, as we have reviewed in detail in earlier chapters, the biologists in the Darwinian tradition prefer to imagine many intergrading "steps" in the accumulation of large-scale phenotypic change. And there is a persistent, if seldom emphasized, theme in Darwinian-based macroevolutionary theory: the concept of *Stufenreihen*, in which continua of accumulating adaptive change are seen occurring in a series of more or less discrete steps.

Simpson (1944, p. 194; 1953, p. 220) explicitly introduced the German term *Stufenreihe* (literally, "series of steps") into the evolutionary discourse of the synthesis. He utilized the concept to explain his vision of how shifts between "adaptive zones" might be accomplished. Each step represents invasion of a stable subzone between the two major adaptive zones, one the zone from which the lineage begins, and the other the zone which comes to be occupied by transformation of some of the members of the ancestral lineage.

Occupation of the intermediate subzones is not necessarily transitory; Simpson imagined a variegated pattern of persistence and ex-

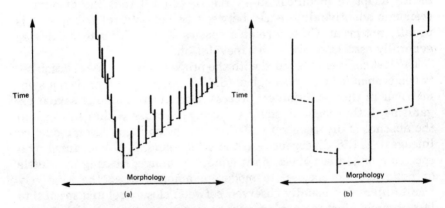

Figure 5.1 Diagram comparing rates of morphological change and rates of speciation. Comparable degrees of phenotypic change over the same interval of time are portrayed in (*a*) and (*b*). In (*a*), the change is accrued through many speciation events, each entailing relatively small amounts of phenotypic change; in (*b*), fewer speciation events, each entailing relatively larger amounts of morphological change than in the speciation events in (*a*), result in a total accrual of within-lineage evolutionary change comparable to that seen in (*a*).

tinction through time. In the long run, however, most of the intermediate subzones would be vacated through extinction, leaving only
living members of the ancestral and derived adaptive zones and perhaps (erroneously) fostering the impression that intermediates between the organisms occupying the two zones in fact never existed.

Bock (1965, see Chap. 3) utilized such a model in his exploration of
the origin of avian flight; his later work (e.g., 1979) more explicitly
linked the intermediate subzones with speciation itself. More recently
other biologists (e.g., Futuyma, 1987) have seen speciation as a means
of injecting economic adaptive change into the phylogenetic history of
lineages; successive speciations can act to accumulate such change
through time. There is something of a consensus emerging among
macroevolutionists in general that speciation acts like a "ratchet":
change is both conserved and fostered by the speciation process itself.
When speciation occurs, whatever economic adaptive change is associated with it becomes available as the starting point for further adaptive change in the phylogenetic future. The metaphor of the ratchet
carries the further implication of inherent directionality: change
tends to accumulate in one direction only—it cannot "go back" to some
former state. As we review the various models implicating speciation
with macroevolution, some will indeed consider such a possibility of
"directional" phenotypic change associated with speciation, while others will not insist on such a tight causal link between speciation and
direction of economic adaptive change. Most recent models of "species
selection" and "species sorting" focus primarily on the role of differential rates of production of new species (speciation) and their disappearance (extinction) as a component of change in the genetic variance
available at any one time for (1) the stocking of economic systems (ecosystems) and (2) further evolutionary change. To evaluate these models accurately, we must first consider in somewhat greater detail exactly what manner of entities species really *are*.

The Role of Species in Nature

Wright (1931, 1932) pictured species as distributed into a number of
subcomponents, which he called "semi-isolated colonies" and later
simply "demes." As we have seen, Dobzhansky (1937*a* and many later
references) adopted this view of the structure of species completely.
Both he and Wright before him saw the significance of such structure
as perhaps best favoring continuing evolutionary change: the semi-
independence of the colonies would allow the accumulation of partly
independent evolutionary histories through both natural selection
and Wright's concept of genetic drift. On the other hand, a species

composed of many such colonies would not run the risk of depleting its total amount of genetic variance, a factor also important in long-range evolutionary activity.

There is little doubt that Wright's picture of species' structure is generally accurate and holds for the vast majority of species. No species is distributed uniformly over its entire range. This is obviously so for those distributed over dramatically patchy terrain, where suitable habitat is interrupted (forming "islands") by vast stretches of totally unsuitable environments. Islands, mountaintops, and the rock kopjes of eastern and southern Africa are all graphic examples: klipspringers (African antelope, the species *Oreotragus oreotragus*) are confined to the rock kopjes, separated by vast seas of (for them) uninhabitable grassy plains or scrub.

Yet all species exhibit some degree of heterogeneity in their distributions. Even vast, fairly uniform geographical stretches of environment are irregularly populated by members of any given species, either because of microvariation in the distribution of resources or essentially random factors of colonization and local extinction. We have already explored one major implication of this structure of (partial) discontinuity between local populations within a species: the semi-independent histories of such colonies militates against a concerted specieswide direction in accumulation of adaptive change through time. Though the opportunity for continued evolutionary change on the local level is perhaps enhanced through such structure, the development of semi-isolated subdivisions of a species has the effect of specieswide net stasis, in which little in the way of specieswide long-term economic adaptive change is likely to accumulate.

We now examine this structure of species—divided as most are into a series of partly isolated populations—from a slightly different angle. We need to know, in particular, what the nature of these subunits is. Recalling the two great classes of organismic behavior (or of biological activity in general), we can ask if species and their component, local populations are either genealogical in nature (that is, tied to the reproductive activities of organisms), or whether they are economic systems of some sort (i.e., arising out of the economic adaptations of organisms), or whether species and their subdivisions can reasonably be viewed as both sorts of entities. The issue is critical, because much of macroevolutionary theory sees species (and higher taxa) as economic entities. We need to know what taxa are, i.e., what role(s) they play in nature, before we can assess their function in evolution.

In Chap. 4, we reviewed a spectrum of opinion on what manner of entity species might be construed to be. To the extent that they are seen as real spatiotemporally bounded entities, species are nearly always taken to be primarily *reproductive communities*. And, especially if Paterson's (1985) views are followed, species arise strictly out of the reproductive behaviors of organisms, and the ongoing (sexual) selection for continued mate recognition and successful mating. Thus species are reproductive (genealogical) entities; but this conclusion by no means implies that species cannot be, in some sense, economic entities as well.

And that is precisely the way some evolutionists have seen species: as economic entities. Dobzhansky (1951), in the passage quoted earlier in this book (p. 19), a passage that sets the dominant theme for macroevolution under the synthesis, speaks of species as having "niches." More recently, Mayr (1982a, p. 273) has added the occupation of niches as a property in his very definition of the term "species." And while much confusion has permeated the concept of niche within ecology as well as in evolutionary biology, there is no question that niches are generally construed as *components of economic (ecological) systems.*

When ecologists refer to niches—even to the niche of certain, particular species—the context is invariably local ecosystems. Niches of yellow-headed blackbirds in a marsh in Iowa may be described and compared with niches of other species in the same ecosystem, or with yellow-headed blackbirds in other ecosystems elsewhere. Only in the rare situation when a species has dwindled to the size of a single local population does an ecologist speak of the niche and mean the niche *of an entire species.*

Damuth (1985) has coined the useful term "avatar" for local populations of a species integrated into a particular ecosystem or ecological community. Avatars are seen as actual *parts* of such local ecosystems. Thus it is avatars, rather than species, that have ecological niches. Because species are, as a rule, distributed into more than one local ecosystem, there are many local avatars, hence localized niches, within any species. Crucial to macroevolutionary theory, then, is the question: Can we sum up local avatars and speak of a specieswide niche? Further, can we sum up the niches of closely related species within higher, monophyletic taxa (Chap. 6) and speak of the niches (or "adaptive zones") of higher taxa?

Because monophyletic taxa consist of one (and usually many more) species, any characterization of the economic role played by species also holds true for monophyletic taxa. We have already hinted at the confusion that naturally arises when considering niches of species: because local populations of a single species (avatars) are commonly regarded as parts of local economic systems (ecosystems), and because they are referred to as "species X" and "species Y" in the ecological literature, there has been little hesitation within biology in general to consider species as having niches.

The idea that species have niches (and that monophyletic taxa occupy adaptive zones) stems from the observation that most members of a species (regardless of where, and in what ecological setting, they occur) as a rule tend to resemble one another more closely than they do members of other species. And, as we have already seen, most of the close resemblance among members of a single species involves economic adaptive features of the phenotype. Thus, although there is some geographical variation (especially in average adult size) in local populations of coyotes (*Canis latrans*), members of the species share a phenotypic resemblance that clearly stamps them as coyotes wherever they may occur in North America. Moreover, though coyotes are found in a rather wide range of habitats (from the deserts of the southwest to the forests of the northeast), there is a certain behavioral repertoire that stamps them as coyotes wherever they occur. Thus, wherever they occur, and no matter how different their habitats, prey items, etc., may be from place to place, coyotes are found to be performing a familiar, rather similar economic role. It is because of this sameness (with local variations) in the sorts of ecological roles played by local populations of species (avatars) that most biologists are comfortable with the notion that species as a whole have niches.

Yet, for entire species to have niches in the same sense that avatars have niches, species would have to be demonstrable parts of actual biological economic systems, ecosystems on some scale larger than the local systems composed of different avatars. And this is precisely where some authors (Eldredge and Salthe, 1984; Eldredge, 1985a, 1986) have criticized conventional wisdom that sees species as occupying niches. The problem is best approached by comparing the distributions of species, on the one hand, with the distributions of ecosystems (or, more simply, habitats). Although ecologists differ strongly among themselves about the discreteness, even the "reality," of ecological systems,[1] no one disagrees that there is energy flow and matter–energy transfer between organisms *of different species* that can be observed on the local level, virtually anywhere at any time. No matter how vague the boundaries between local systems, such systems clearly exist and are linked laterally (geographically) with other such systems to form more regional biotal systems.

Maps of species distribution simply do not conform to the map of ecosystem distribution over the same areal extent. Whereas ecosystems are linked into spatially adjoining systems to form regional economic systems, a single species tends to be represented within some habitats locally and not found in other, adjacent habitats within the larger ecological system. Instead, species are often distributed in (suitable) habitats in *other* economic systems. A single species may have representatives (avatars) in a number of quite different ecosystems, a point

Vrba (1988) makes clearly in conjunction with her analysis of the distribution of modern populations of the African buffalo *Syncerus caffer*. Put another way, the total geographic distribution of any given species (unless it exists only as a single avatar) ordinarily does not conform to the distributional limits of mappable ecosystems. A map of current coyote distribution in North America does *not* yield simultaneously a map of a single, complex megaecosystem. The point is made even clearer if we examine the distributions of the prey items of coyotes throughout their ranges. Though some species of jackrabbits may have coyotes distributed throughout their ranges, cottontails and snowshoe hares are distributed more widely than are coyotes—yet are coyote food items when their ranges do overlap. The point is simply that a map of ecosystems based on rabbits yields an entirely different ecological picture than one based on coyote distribution.

We can only conclude that species, *as entire entities,* simply are not parts of specifiable, mappable economic systems. Species as composite wholes therefore do not have niches—at least in the same sense that local populations of conspecifics (avatars) are said to have niches. Rather, from an ecological (economic) point of view, species have a no less important, but rather different, significance. Wherever they occur, members of a spcies perform *analogous* economic roles. There is variation, of course: lions in southern Africa (Namib desert), for example, have developed a method of stalking and killing oryxes (gemsbok) that is not used on similar species elsewhere in Africa. Yet the general role of lions as top predator is basically similar wherever lions occur. But rather than speaking of the "niche of the species lion" (as Dobzhansky does in his famous passage on macroevolution), a preferable description of nature is to see redundancy in the nature of the actual, realized niches of local avatars of *Felis leo*.

Wright, in developing his picture of species divided up into semiautonomous "local colonies," later called these subdivisions "demes." As we have seen, Damuth prefers the term "avatars" to describe local manifestations of a species playing a particular role in a local ecosystem. "Deme," however, remains a useful term; it has been used by some authors (e.g., Eldredge and Salthe, 1984) specifically to refer to local breeding populations of species. That is to say, if species are reproductive communities (as developed in the preceding chapter) arising from the sexual reproductive behaviors of their component organisms, then, since species are distributed discontinuously, there must be local subdivisions into reproductive populations. The term "deme" remains convenient for such local breeding populations of conspecifics. The possibility that local avatars and demes are in fact coextensive (or nearly so), so that at least at times within some species locally, avatars and demes may be one and the same thing, is briefly considered further below. But the distinction between avatars and demes is not merely conceptual: very often, local economic populations (avatars) are not the same as demes. Bull elephants, for example, spend most of the year off on their own, while cows and immatures form hierarchically structured social groups.

Thus, a sharper picture of what species *are* seems to be emerging: species are reproductive communities composed of organisms sharing a single fertilization system; they are distributed discontinuously; and their component organisms play analogous economic roles in different local ecosystems. Local avatars of species perform direct economic roles. From an economic point of view, however, species in their entirety play no concerted role as parts of single, large-scale systems. They are, instead, largely redundant packages of genetic information—information, moreover, that is mostly concerned with the economic adaptations of organisms. It is this retention of largely redundant genetic information on economic adaptations that (of course) underlies the morphological and behavioral similarities between widely distributed avatars and leads especially to the similar economic roles played by members of avatars of the same species wherever they occur. But this redundancy has also led to the mistaken impression that species as a whole have ecological niches.

Now, in turning to the several aspects of the debate over "species selection," we will see why an accurate grasp of the nature of species— the role(s) species actually play in nature—is important to modern macroevolutionary theory.

Species Sorting and Species Selection: General Considerations

Whatever their precise nature may be, species have come to be regarded by many biologists as *spatiotemporally bounded entities* (Chap. 4). This means, simply, that species have origins (speciation), histories, and, ultimately, terminations (extinctions). That species have histories may come as no surprise, yet a curious implication of the biological species concept to Mayr (e.g., 1988) and Bock (e.g., 1979) is that species *do not* exist in any real sense through time. Nonetheless, a prevalent theme in modern evolutionary theory sees species as real entities that exist for nontrivial lengths of geological time.

Because monophyletic taxa typically consist of many (often thousands of) species, and because species become extinct as well as (from time to time) giving rise to new descendant species, the species composition of higher taxa is expected, in the very nature of things, to change through time. Patterns of species stability and change within monophyletic taxa have come to be a major theme in contemporary macroevolutionary theory. And the search for causal pathways underlying such stability and change—the topic of "species sorting" and "species selection"—has proven (to some extent unnecessarily) to be one of the more controversial topics in evolutionary biology.

Yet there is more than a general expectation that species composition of monophyletic taxa will change through time: the fossil record bears dramatic and even obvious evidence that such is the case. No species of marine invertebrate found in Devonian strata is known to exist today—implying that hard-shelled invertebrate species of the mid-Paleozoic are now all extinct *and* that hard-shelled invertebrates in modern seas evolved at some time later than the Paleozoic. Coming closer to the Recent, examination of Cretaceous mollusks (by this time many of the modern families of clams and snails had already appeared) shows that the composition of these families on the generic and species level was different from that observed today.

The idea that there may be biological factors biasing the "births and deaths" of species within monophyletic taxa had a more specific origin as a corollary to the development of punctuated equilibria. As Eldredge and Gould (1972, p. 111) pointed out, the observation that most species do not accrue substantial amounts of new directional adaptive change during the course of their history (the phenomenon of *stasis*—Chap. 4) poses something of a paradox: If natural selection is *not* constantly working at the modification of the economic adaptations of organisms, how then can we explain the directionality evident in the evolutionary history of some sets of morphological features known to have occurred during the phylogenetic histories of some lineages? In other words, we know there have been evolutionary trends in the histories of some taxa; yet, if the history of the individual, component species of these lineages is more one of stability than one of directional change, how are such trends produced?

Hence the paradox: traditional Darwinian-based evolutionary theory has no difficulty explaining long-term evolutionary trends. As Darwin himself argued (especially by analogy with artificial breeding), the degree of morphological change that can be effected via short-term selection may reasonably be expected to be magnified proportionately through the passage of time on a geological scale. Small amounts of change accrue over relatively brief intervals; larger intervals simply produce greater amounts of change. The concept of punctuated equilibria, on the other hand, based as it is on the empirical generalization that within-species phylogenetic history is seldom unidirectionally anagenetic, eliminates the convenient, traditional Darwinian model of directional macroevolutionary change.

We will consider macroevolutionary patterns in taxic diversity—and their relation to patterns of accumulation of adaptive morphological change—fully in Chap. 6. We consider trends here, however, because of their close association with the development of the debate on species selection, and because the accumulation of (largely) directional adaptive change lies at the very heart of evolutionary theory since its very inception. Directionality, whether or not considered alongside "improvement," has always been a central theme in evolutionary biology.

First, we must consider briefly the very real possibility that directionality itself has been overstated, or at least overemphasized, in evolutionary biology. After all, there is nothing obviously directional about the change in species (and higher-level monophyletic taxon) composition between the Devonian and Recent macroinvertebrate shelly faunas. Nor would it be evident to anyone comparing gastropod shells of the Cretaceous and Recent that there has been a net *direction* (let alone an obvious "improvement") in gastropod shell architecture over the past 65 million years. Some authors have pointed out (Eldredge and Gould, 1972; Eldredge, 1985a) that many "trends" singled out by evolutionary biologists are ex post facto renderings of phylogenetic history: biologists may simply pick out species at different points in geological time that seem to fit on some line of directional modification through time. Many trends, in other words, may exist more in the minds of the analysts than in phylogenetic history. This is particularly so in situations, especially common prior to about 1970, in which analysis of the phylogenetic relationships among species was incompletely or poorly done (see Chap. 6).

Even when trends are real (i.e., reflecting an actual directional change of state within a system), perceptual error in characterization of the trend may lead to incorrect analysis of underlying cause. Gould (1988) has discussed this problem in detail, showing that many "trends" reflect simple change in variance. His most graphic example is the decline of the .400 hitter in baseball, which "is not the gradual extinction of a valued 'thing,' " but is rather the result of an overall improvement in level of play: higher standards have caused a symmetrical decrease in variance of batting averages. The number of players with batting averages lower than .200 has declined as markedly as has the number of averages greater than .400. Gould (1988) argues that much the same sort of phenomenon holds for macroevolutionary trends, many of which may be more appropriately attributed to change in diversity of species in subclades within higher taxa than to a process of anagenetic, directional change through time.

With the caveat that many supposed evolutionary trends are artifacts of analysis firmly in mind, it is important to stress at this juncture that trends—directional accumulations of (presumably) adaptive change—are nonetheless very much a real phenomenon of evolutionary history. Nor need we rely strictly on the fossil record for empirical verification that this must be so. Consider, as a rather striking example met in passing in Chap. 2, the evolutionary history of both absolute and relative brain size (i.e., relative to body size) in hominid evolution. The average cranial capacity of modern *Homo sapiens* is something on the order of 1400 cc, with notable amounts of sexual, geographic, and simple within-population variation. Average cranial capacities for living great apes are considerably less: for example, 400 cc for chimpanzees (*Pan troglodytes*) and 500 cc for gorillas (*Gorilla gorilla*). Thus regardless of which of the competing schemes of phylogenetic relationships for these taxa we accept,[2] we know that there must have been an increase in brain size since the point at which our species (i.e., *H. sapiens*) last shared a common ancestry with one of the extant species of great ape. We would predict, therefore, that there would be a trend towards increase in brain size in the fossilized skulls of members of our own phylogenetic lineage since the point of phylogenetic separation from the great apes.

The fossil record of human evolution amply bears out the predicted pattern of increase in brain size through time. Cranial capacities of the early australopithecine species *Australopithecus africanus* average around 450 cc, hardly to be distinguished from the values for modern-day great apes. Especially within our own, gracile sublineage, i.e., through *Homo habilis* and the later *H. erectus* (see Fig. 5.2), it is clear that mean brain size increases through time. There is no doubt that the trend—which we know from the principles of comparative morphology *must* have occurred—really in fact *did* occur.

Yet it is the precise pattern of increase in brain size which nicely illustrates a central theoretical dispute in macroevolutionary theory.

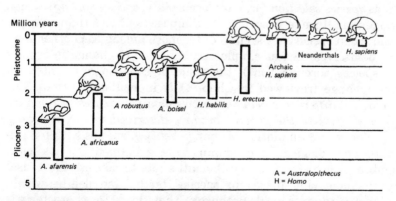

Figure 5.2   The trend towards increase in cranial capacity (brain size) within hominids is evident in the fossil record, whether the record is interpreted in a gradual, or (as here) in a more "punctuated," pattern. (Based on an original diagram by Nicholas Amorosi for Eldredge and Tattersall, 1982)

Paleoanthropologists have for the most part tended to interpret human evolution as a matter of more or less linear transformation of a single lineage through time. In so doing, of course, they have simply been echoing tendencies prevalent in evolutionary paleontology (and evolutionary biology in general) since the nineteenth century. More recently, however, a combination of empirical evidence and reanalysis of existing material has demonstrated partial overlap in temporal occurrence of distinctly different hominids—pointing to the existence of more than one species of hominid alive at any one time. For example, *Homo erectus* and a member of the "robust" lineage of australopithecines are now known to have coexisted during an interval in eastern Africa.

With the recent tendency to interpret the hominid fossil record in terms of a number of species whose spatiotemporal distributions may, in fact, sometimes overlap has come an examination of morphological change *within* species through time. Some paleoanthropologists have argued that there is considerable stasis even in brain size evolution throughout considerable segments of time. Because there is stratigraphic overlap between some species, these anthropologists have raised the possibility that brain size increase in human evolution is at least partly a matter of *species sorting:* rather than there being a linear, progressive increase in brain size through time within a single lineage, or even simply periods of little or no change interrupting briefer periods where change does occur, it is possible to see brain size increase in human evolution as at least partly a matter of larger-brained species outlasting smaller-brained taxa and giving rise to still later species with still bigger brains.

And that is the stark contrast between traditional Darwinian-based explanation of evolutionary trends and the general category of notions known as *species selection* (or, more accurately, *species sorting*). When a phylogenetic lineage is seen to be composed of more than one species, and when species are seen to differ more among each other than *within* themselves (i.e., as simple accumulation of change internally within species through time), the issue of evolutionary context of adaptive change (reviewed in Chap. 4) is immediately raised. *The morphological differences between species as a rule represent adaptive change and arise in the general manner described in the preceding chapter.* Yet the accumulation of change *between* species within a lineage through geological time remains to be explained. Species selection embraces a body of theory that attempts to address the causal pathways underlying biases in species' births and deaths within monophyletic taxa—causal pathways that lead to characteristic macroevolutionary patterns such as evolutionary trends. Contrary to some characterizations, species selection is by no means an alternative causal theory of the origin of organismic adaptations; it *is* an attempt to refine understanding of the patterns of distribution of such adaptations through phylogenetic history. If species really do function as "ratchets" in the accumulation of large-scale adaptive change (macroevolution) the phenomenon of species sorting (whether or not it is properly termed species selection) is a vital dynamic process determining the actual nature and patterns of phylogenetic accumulations of adaptive change. And the point of departure for all discussions of species selection is always the recognition that species are spatio-temporally bounded entities, linked in complex genealogical patterns to form monophyletic taxa of higher categorical rank.

Species Selection: Definition and Criteria for Recognition

S. M. Stanley (1975) introduced the term "species selection" to embrace the patterns of differential species births and deaths discussed in the original paper on punctuated equilibria (Eldredge and Gould, 1972). Stanley (1975, p. 648) made the explicit analogy between natural selection and species selection:

> If most evolutionary change occurs during speciation events and if speciation events are largely random, natural selection, long viewed as the process of guiding evolutionary change, cannot play a significant role in determining the overall course of evolution. Macroevolution is decoupled from microevolution, and we must envision the process governing its course as being analogous to natural selection but operating at a higher level of biological organization. In this higher-level process species become analogous to individuals, and speciation replaces reproduction (Table 1) [reproduced here as Table 5.1]. The random aspects of speciation take the place of mutation. Whereas natural selection operates upon individuals within populations, a process that can be termed *species selection* operates upon species within higher taxa, determining statisti-

TABLE 5.1   Stanley's Comparison of Analogous Features of Natural Selection and Species Selection

Process	Unit of selection	Source of variability	Type of selection
Microevolution	Individual	Mutation, recombination	Natural selection A. Survival vs. death B. Rate of reproduction
Macroevolution	Species	Speciation	Species selection A. Survival vs. extinction B. Rate of speciation

SOURCE: From Stanley (1975) Table 1, p. 649.

cal trends. In natural selection types of individuals are favored that tend to (A) survive to reproduction age and (B) exhibit high fecundity. The two comparable traits of species selection are (A) survival for long periods, which increases chances of speciation and (B) tendency to speciate at high rates. Extinction, of course, replaces death in the analogy.

Though, as Stanley pointed out, biologists as far back as Darwin had occasionally depicted evolution as a "race among evolving species," species selection, seen as a process analogous to natural selection but "operating at a higher level of biological organization" (as Stanley puts it) has served as the focal point for all subsequent discussions within macroevolutionary theory—and served, as well, as a major impetus for the development of theories of the hierarchical structure of biological systems and their role in the evolutionary process (see Chaps. 6 and 7 for more on hierarchy theory).

Species-selection theory is still in its relative infancy. In general, evolutionary biologists focusing on patterns of generation-by-generation change in gene frequencies naturally have rather little use for the concept of among-species sorting. Some (e.g., Maynard Smith, 1987; see also Thompson, 1983) see species selection as an alternative model for the origin of organismic adaptations and have little difficulty in rejecting the notion altogether as nonsensical. Others (e.g., Dawkins, 1986) grasp the basic ideas accurately, but claim that species selection, largely because it works over such long temporal scales, cannot possibly be as important a determinant of evolutionary patterns as natural selection, which works, of course, on a generation-by-generation basis. Other evolutionary biologists (as we have seen to some extent already in Chaps. 2 and 3) are beginning to incorporate patterns of among-species evolutionary stasis and change with the more familiar within-species phenomena.

Yet, for the most part, it is paleontologists (and, to a lesser extent, systematists) who have developed and debated species selection, simply because the data of paleontology are at the proper scale for analyzing patterns of differential species births and deaths within monophyletic taxa through time. E. S. Vrba (1980, 1984a; Vrba and Eldredge 1984; Vrba and Gould, 1986; and other publications) has been especially active in exploring the nature of species selection as a process occurring at the "higher level of organization" that species represent and as a process originally depicted to be a strict analogue of natural selection. When various competing claims on species selection are reviewed, it quickly becomes clear that theoretical distinctions between various forms of species selection and between species selection and other possible causal pathways underlying patterns of differential species production and survival are relatively easy to enumerate. Far more difficult is determining which models apply to specific cases of phylogenetic history.

There is an important distinction, first, to be drawn between *species sorting,* the general term for patterns of differential births and deaths of species within monophyletic taxa, and *species selection,* which, however defined, is a theory of causation underlying such sorting. The point is—as Vrba and Eldredge (1984) and especially Vrba and Gould (1986) have argued—there are several possible causes in addition to species selection which may underlie a given instance of species sorting. In particular, the causal mechanism underlying sorting may occur *at the level of species,* or might arise, instead, *from another (lower) level.* Only the former is properly construed as species selection (Vrba, 1980); where causation of species sorting arises from lower (i.e., organismic or genic) levels, Vrba (1980) speaks of the *effect hypothesis* (see below) rather than species selection.

The conclusion that causal mechanisms must operate directly at a given level for selection to be said to occur at that level follows particularly clearly from a general analysis of the nature of *all* selection by Hull (1980). Hull was concerned with evaluating the presence of selection at various different levels of biological organization. To do so, he presented a two-part criterion serving as both the definition and the basis of recognition of selection at any level. Hull wrote (1980, p. 318):

> ...the two sorts of entities that function in selection processes can be defined as follows:
>
> *replicator:* an entity that passes on its structure directly in replication, and
>
> *interactor:* an entity that directly interacts as a cohesive whole with its environment in such a way that replication is differential.
>
> With the aid of these two technical terms, the selection process itself can be defined:
>
> *selection:* a process in which the differential extinction and proliferation of interactors cause the differential perpetuation of the replicators that produced them.

With Hull's characterization of *replicators* and *interactors* in mind, let us briefly look at Darwinian natural selection as a paradigm example of what selection is (and recalling that Stanley originally framed his characterization of species selection as an exact analogue of natural selection). Organisms are both interactors and reproducers, with underlying replicative fidelity supplied at the genomic level. Organismic selection arises from differential (economic) success of conspecific organisms within local populations (avatars): on average, organisms carrying traits that confer relatively greater economic (interactive) success will have a higher probability of reproductive success than less economically successful members of the local deme.

In this, the original Darwinian version of natural selection, both the interacting and the reproducing are done by organisms within larger-scale entities (local avatars and demes). It is true that actual *replication* of genetic information takes place at a lower level—in higher organisms, within nuclei and mitochondria (or chloroplasts) of cells of the germ line. But this must be the case for all levels of selection. For selection to occur at levels other than genes themselves, we must modify Hull's formulation a bit: *both interaction and reproduction ("moremaking" of entities of like kind) must occur within a single category of entity at a given level for selection truly analogous to natural selection to be said to occur at levels higher (or lower) than the organismic level.*

By this modified version of Hull's criteria for recognizing selection, it is immediately apparent that species selection cannot be fully analogous to natural selection, because species themselves are not interactors. Species are not parts of economic systems, and do not interact as whole entities either with the physical environment or with other entities, such as other species.[3]

But species do "reproduce," i.e., species, by speciation, give rise to entities of like kind: descendant species. As Stanley (1975) pointed out, speciation is directly analogous to reproduction in asexual organisms. And, because we might anticipate there to be factors systematically biasing birth and death rates of species within monophyletic taxa, it follows that were selection to occur at the level of species, such species selection might be most properly considered analogous to sexual selection. Yet there is interaction in Darwin's original concept of sexual selection, which he defined as the advantage some organisms of the same sex and species enjoy over others purely in relation to ability to reproduce successfully. For species selection to be demonstrated, the factors biasing species birth and death rates would have to be shown to derive from properties of a species (just as both forms of organismic selection derive from properties held by organisms); and for the analogy to hold with force, we might also expect there to be some form of interaction among species, if not economic (ecological), then at least in terms of competition for "speciation success."

Thus there are two rather severe conceptual difficulties in characterizing *species* selection as a direct, higher-level analogue of *natural* selection. First, species cannot realistically be described as interactors—certainly not in the same sense in which we see organisms as interactors. Secondly, for the analogy to hold, we would expect species selection to arise from properties *of species,* just as (Darwinian, eco-

nomic) natural selection represents the sorting of phenotypic properties *of organisms*. This latter point merits further comment.

The original formulations of species selection in macroevolutionary
theory (i.e., Eldredge and Gould, 1972; Stanley, 1975) were concerned
with patterns of stasis and change *in the distribution of organismic
phenotypic attributes*. Species selection, in other words, was propounded to supply additional needed causal theory to explain patterns
of organismic phenotype distributions within phylogenetic histories.
The "trends" singled out for special attention, for example, all involved phenotypic characteristics of organisms. The original problem,
as stated both by Eldredge and Gould (1972) and by Stanley (1975),
was to understand how the directionality of trends could be understood as at least partly an among-species phenomenon: stasis within
species having effectively removed the easy, linear model of long-term
natural selection as the sole causative agent necessary to explain
long-term evolutionary trends. Yet, because *natural* selection deals
with organismic properties, logically *species* selection should deal
with—and, more critically, arise from—species-level properties.

Vrba (1980) was the first to make this distinction clear. Much of the
literature on species selection subsequent to her paper represents attempts to examine the issue of the existence of species-level properties
(or so-called *emergent* properties of species). It must be emphasized
that, to date, there is still a considerable amount of disagreement over
emergence: some authors believe there are such species-level properties, while others remain skeptical. The issue hinges to a significant
extent on the status of organismic attributes distributed specieswide,
and on the notion of frequency distributions of organismic properties
within species. Some evolutionary biologists, going as far back at least
as Dobzhansky (1937a), emphatically feel that frequency distributions
are group-level properties (whether it is demes or entire species that
are the groups—or indeed, whether the groups are higher monophyletic taxa: all mammals have hair, for example). Arnold and
Fristrup (1982), echoing a common theme in the *levels of selection* literature, argue that population structures that arise from peculiarities
of organismic biology are nonetheless group-level traits that bias the
probabilities of both continued existence and reproduction of such entities.

There is no doubt that frequencies of (organismic phenotypic) traits
occupy a somewhat intermediate position between simple organismic
traits varying within a local population, and truly *emergent* properties
of entire groups of organisms. In other words, many biologists (and
philosophers of biology; see Lloyd, 1988) are content to accept as avatar selection the situation in which two disjunct avatars of the same
species suffer different fates in the face of an environmental challenge

strictly because all the organisms of one of the avatars possess one trait not present (or present in an alternative form) in the other avatar. If two species were each reduced to single avatars, such a situation could be accepted as species selection.

Such a loose construction of species selection—in which species (or avatar) sorting arises because of the frequency distributions of organismic phenotypic properties—clearly does not constitute an exact analogue with natural selection. And a deeper issue lurks in such examples of frequency distribution as putative group-level properties: We must ask what the actual dynamics of causal process really are in such situations. Can we attribute the death of one population because of *its* frequency distribution of organismic traits, and the survival of another based on its differing distribution, to a group-level process? Or do we simply have local extinction (natural selection in perhaps its most graphic and sweeping form) extending to wipe out one local population but not the other? In other words, how are we to distinguish, even purely conceptually, between disappearance through the simple summation of the deaths of individuals (selection at the organismic, within-population level) and disappearance because of the high (100 percent) frequency of a nonviable phenotypic property? It does not seem to me overly "reductionist" to see such instances as simple natural selection that have higher, group-level effects—a conclusion argued by Vrba and Eldredge (1984) at length (see Fig. 5.3).

Are there, then, any cases of genuinely specieswide properties that are truly *properties of species rather than simple frequency distributions of organismic properties?* The general picture we have developed so far of the nature of species sees them as characteristically divided up into a number of semi-isolated "colonies" (to use Wright's original term). Whether we view these local groups as avatars (i.e., in an ecological sense) or as demes (as local reproductive communities), local populations within a species are largely redundant on one another. In other words, species are not like well-differentiated entities—in the same sense that an organism can be viewed as an integrated whole composed of many different parts. Separately, the parts of an organism generally do not function; integrated into a soma, they are the parts of a coherent, functional whole. Species, on the other hand, are not that way at all: extinction of some local demes within a species has little if any effect on other conspecific local demes elsewhere.

That species are not like machines with well-differentiated components (the way organisms are) derives from their status as packages of genetic information rather than as interactive parts of ecosystems. In the present context, it suggests that there is little intrinsic about species that we can characterize usefully as *emergent properties.* Vrba (1984a) refers to the phenotypic properties of organisms in general as

Geographic polymorphism in Cepaea

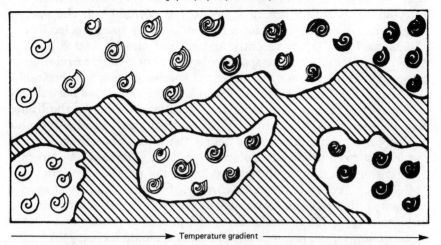

→ Temperature gradient ────────────────────────────→

Figure 5.3 Vrba and Eldredge's example (1984) illustrating differences between "species selection" and "species sorting." The original caption reads: "Deterministic group sorting, because of differences between groups, is not necessarily group selection. In this simple example of shell-banding polymorphism in the snail *Cepaea nemoralis* selection maintains a cline along a temperature gradient. The cline is continuous at the top but interrupted (by unfavorable habitat) into groups at the bottom of the drawing. Local environmental selection in response to temperature change may result in differential group death and birth. But such group sorting results entirely by upward causation from lower-level selection." (Redrawn from Vrba and Eldredge, 1984, Fig. 1, p. 158)

emergent from the level of the genotype. But the functional unity that is an organism is also, if less dramatically, emergent in the sense that component tissues and organs of organisms must all be present, function, and mutually interact in complex ways for the organism itself to be said to exist. And this is precisely what seems to be missing with species in general—properties intrinsic to species that "emerge" as a result of the interactions of its component parts.

There is, however, an exception to the generalization that species lack emergent properties. Paterson's (1985) concept of the SMRS entails interactions between properties of two distinct classes of organisms within species: males and females. By definition, each species has its own unique SMRS. It makes sense, therefore, to conceive of the SMRS as a specieswide property, thus bolstering the conclusion that species selection is the proper analogue of *sexual*—as opposed to *natural*—selection.[4]

And there is a further, major exception to the conclusion that species lack emergent properties in any meaningful sense. There are *extrinsic* features of biological systems, namely, their distribution in space and time. Spatiotemporal location of a species is unique to each species, as is the density and manner of distribution of its component demes–avatars. If it could be shown that aspects of distribution and internal organization are to some degree heritable on the species level, a case could be made for a form of genuine species selection.

Jablonski (1987) has recently argued that closely related pairs of Upper Cretaceous mollusk species display such a high correlation in geographic ranges that areal extent of species is, in effect, heritable. Jablonski (1987, p. 362, Table 2) compared the calculated heritability of the species ranges with other heritabilities culled from the literature on quantitative genetics. That Cretaceous gastropod geographic ranges have heritability values nearly twice that of cattle milk yield (which has been artificially selected for so long) strengthens the possibility that selection at the species level may well be occurring.

Geographic range is inversely correlated with probability of species extinction (for reasons examined more fully in later sections; see Jablonski 1986, 1987). Jablonski (1987, p. 362) concludes that, "other factors being equal, mean geographic range should increase through a clade's history because widespread species are extinction-resistant and tend to give rise to similarly widespread species."

Further, and of potentially more direct relevance to the issues of macroevolutionary stasis and change in organismic phenotypic features, is the possibility of inadvertent "hitchhiking" of organismic traits along with selection at the species level. In particular, those aspects of organismic biology that lead to widespread dispersal are expected to be directly selected—though Jablonski (1987) cites Stanley (1986) to the effect that larval dispersal ability in eastern Pacific Neogene bivalves is *not* correlated with geographic range. But, in addition, there might well be other aspects that are simply correlated with, rather than contributing causal elements of, geographic range that might show differential spread within a clade as a side effect of selection for range size itself; such hitchhiking would be different in basic nature from the species-level "drift" effects expected for non-correlated characters (whether organismic or not).

But even though one might agree that spatiotemporal localization (such as geographic areal extent) qualifies as a heritable and species-level emergent character, thus posing a possibly valid example of true species selection, there is no doubt that such distributions arise in the greatest part from the behaviors and physiologies of the organisms within the species. By far the simpler explanation of biases of both speciation and extinction rate is to see them as side effects from rather straightforward elements of organismic biology—the basic point of Vrba's *effect hypothesis,* to which we now turn.

The Effect Hypothesis and the Relation of Organismic Properties to Species Sorting

Vrba (1984*a*, p. 322) characterizes her *effect hypothesis* in these very general terms:

> If one can explain sorting among species solely by comparison of characters and dynamics at the levels of organisms and genomes (the effect hypothesis), then there is no need to invoke species selection. The argument amounts to a plea for recognition that not all non-random sorting among species need be caused by selection (see discussion in Vrba and Eldredge, 1984) and for restriction of a hypothesis of species selection to a hypothesis of species aptation.

As we have already seen, Vrba (1980 and later references) was the first to point out that species sorting could arise from selection of emergent species-level properties at the level of species—true species selection. But sorting among species may also arise simply from the "effects" of organismic phenotypic properties on either rate of speciation, rate of species extinction, or both. Her earlier discussions linked aspects of ecological (specifically, niche breadth) theory with rates of speciation, in contrast with some earlier discussions of species selection (wrongly so termed) linking niche breadth theory with rates of species extinction (e.g., Eldredge, 1979; Eldredge and Cracraft, 1980).

In general, earlier discussions of species selection did, as Vrba has emphasized, focus on patterns of differential species extinction, because, as Vrba (1984*a*) has put it, "…the preoccupation with differential species extinction makes sense. It is much easier to visualize that what is 'good for the organism' may also improve species longevity, than that it should improve species reproductive rates." But in adding a consideration of various-level causation to understanding differential rates of production of new species, the general discussion of species selection became rather more complex and departed to some extent from the original purpose of the species-selection discussions associated with punctuated equilibria: the explanation of the relation between patterns of species appearance and disappearance, on the one hand, and the spatiotemporal distribution of organismic phenotypic features on the other.

Put another way: if the problem is to explain a trend, e.g., in brain size in hominids, and the pattern seems at least in part to be interspecific, neither true species selection (on emergent properties) *nor* controls of speciation and extinction rates as a consequence of organismic phenotypic properties can be shown to be causally linked to the production of such a trend *unless the characters "hitchhike" in the manner advocated by Jablonski (1987) for true species selection, or the organismic characters underlying the effect are the same as, or linked to, the characters showing the trend pattern.* This, of course, is a tall order, although it has been approached in some examples. But it must be stressed before reviewing Vrba's original example of the effect hypothesis that first, sorting of species, regardless of cause, is important to macroevolution simply because the "standing crop" of species diversity at any one time provides the basis for the filling of contemporaneous ecosystems, and the basis of all future evolution. Sorting of species changes that basis. But second, species sorting is even more crucial to theories of the macroevolutionary transformation of organismic phenotypes (the central theme of this book) if the characters undergoing macroevolutionary change are implicated more directly—either as cause, or effect, or a mixture of the two—in processes of species-level sorting, which, as we have already seen, can arise in several distinct ways.

Like the earlier discussions of species selection, Vrba's original discussion and examples of *effect macroevolution* are directed at phylogenetic trends. Although her most general statement of effect macroevolution simply sees differential species production (and/or survival) arising as a side effect of any aspect of organismic phenotypic properties, the particular example Vrba chose to illustrate her initial discussion of effect macroevolution (Vrba, 1980) specifically focused on aspects of *niche breadth*. In brief, Vrba (1980; also 1984*b*) has argued that species composed of organisms that are relatively broad niched (*eurytopic*) tend to display lower rates of both speciation and (species-level) extinction than more narrow niched species. Trends develop as a side effect of intrinsically higher rates of speciation in the more narrow niched lineages. The distinction is especially clear in sister lineages in which one lineage remains relatively eurytopic and the other contains more stenotopic species.

Following the discussion in earlier sections of this chapter, it is important to reiterate that it is not species per se that are eurytopic or stenotopic. Fox and Morrow (1981) have discussed the two senses in which species might be considered eurytopic or stenotopic; in neither sense is the species as an entire entity said to be occupying a niche, whether broad or narrow. Rather, eurytopy and stenotopy most commonly refer to the physiological and behavioral aspects of the economic life of individual *organisms*. Some "kinds" of organisms (which is to say, organisms in some species, in contrast to organisms in other species), display greater characteristic tolerances to environmental extremes (salinity, for example, or oxygen tension in an aqueous environment, or temperature). Another common parameter discussed in terms of niche breadth is utilization of food resources. Organisms within some species are able to utilize a greater spectrum of food resources than are organisms from other species; the shorthand way of characterizing such differences is simply to say that species X has a broader niche than species Y. *But the differences really arise strictly from the specieswide distribution of phenotypic properties—especially aspects of physiology and behavior.*

Fox and Morrow (1981) point out that polymorphism within a species can also amount to eurytopy. Thus, eurytopy might arise because of among-organismic variation, in addition to within-organismic breadth of tolerance. In any case, however it arises, eurytopy is not an absolute property: rather eurytopy and stenotopy constitute a sliding scale of relative niche breadth—hence the value of comparing closely related organisms. Moreover, organisms may be relatively broadly tolerant in respect to some parameters and rather narrowly adapted in others. In some species, niche width changes seasonally; in others, relative niche width seems to vary systematically with stages in a life cycle.

With all these caveats, however, correlations of aspects of niche width with species-level diversity and apparent rates of accumulation of evolutionary adaptive change have been documented for many different groups[5]—enough that some generalizations can indeed be made about the effect of niche width on speciation, extinction, and morphological change in evolution. Vrba (1980, 1984b) presents an especially well documented example, which we shall review briefly before examining in greater detail the causal links between niche width and evolution.

Vrba (1980) studied African antelopes of two different clades (lineages): the Aepycerotini (impalas) and Alcelaphini (wildebeests, hartebeests, bonteboks, and kin). Phylogenetic analysis demonstrated close kinship between the two clades, and Vrba concludes that the two subtribes are sister groups.

The two lineages apparently split in the Upper Miocene, some 5 million years ago. Because horn morphology forms part of the SMRS in antelopes, and is readily preserved in the fossil record, it is possible for paleontologists to derive an accurate assessment of the actual number of species within each lineage through time, basing their judgments on the same identification criteria that the organisms themselves use. According to Vrba, there is 1 single, widespread, and geographically variable species of impala extant in the Recent biota; there are 7 species of alcelaphines. During the past 5 million years, there has been a minimum of 25 additional species of alcelaphines, while the record suggests that there have been at most only 2 additional species of impala. In any case, there seems to have been but 1 impala species extant at any one time during the past 5 million years.

Figure 5.4 illustrates Vrba's data for the various fossil and Recent species. Extinction and speciation rates are obviously much higher within the alcelaphines than within the aepycerotines. Species-level diversity, moreover, correlates highly with rates of anatomical transformation. The wildebeests (gnus) are among the most highly derived species of any bovid lineage. The impalas, in contrast, have changed very little from their initial anatomical configuration.[6]

Thus the aepycerotines are species-poor and have changed relatively little since their inception; they have low extinction rates as well. Alcelaphines, on the other hand, are species-rich, showing high rates of speciation and extinction. They have accrued much more mor-

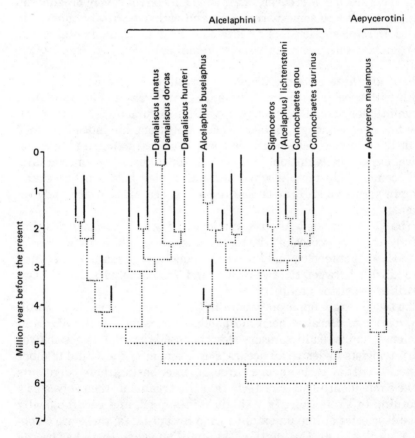

Figure 5.4 Vrba's diagram depicting "different speciation rates in the sister-group Alcelaphini-Aepycerotini. Known species' durations (*solid lines*) arranged in a cladogram against the time scale." (Redrawn from Vrba, 1980, Fig. 13, p. 73)

phological change within the lineage as a whole than has their impala sister lineage. (Gnus are more derived than other extant alcelaphines, such as bonteboks, and show up later in the fossil record than less highly derived species.) This pattern of speciation, extinction, and morphological change, in turn, correlates rather closely with characteristics of niche breadth of organisms within species of the two different sister lineages.

Impalas are notoriously eurytopic. They occur in a wide range of habitats, from open plains to wooded grasslands and even forests. They browse on leaves and graze on grass. Alcelaphines, in contrast, are strictly grazers. Alcelaphines, too, are more narrowly restricted in the range of habitats in which they occur. Greenacre and Vrba (1984) report that, all told, the actual biomass of impalas in any one area (for example, Kruger National Park, South Africa) tends to equal or even slightly surpass the total biomass of all alcelaphines combined. Thus specialization vs. being an ecological generalist has rather different implications not only for "standing crop" of biomass locally, but evidently for long-term speciation, extinction, and accrual of adaptive change. The details of the cases presented by Novacek (1984), Fryer and Iles (1969), and others are closely similar to those of Vrba's antelope example. There seems to be a common recurring association between speciation and extinction rates, which are positively correlated with rate of accumulation of adaptive change and with degree of ecological specialization. Yet there are conflicting interpretations of causal pathways interlinking these different evolutionary parameters.

Rates of Speciation, Extinction, and Morphological Change: The Ecological Link

Vrba (1980) presented the impala–wildebeest contrast in conjunction with her initial discussion of the effect hypothesis. Pointing out (as we have already seen) that earlier discussions of species selection had focused much more attention on differential species persistence (i.e., patterns of extinction) than on causal relations leading to differential speciation per se, Vrba sought to explain the African antelope example (including the trend towards more derived morphology within the alcelaphine, or wildebeest, clade) in terms primarily of differential rates of species production within predominantly stenotopic lineages: higher rates of speciation were held, in particular, to arise from the stenotopic nature of the organisms within the species of the clade.

Vrba (1980, 1984a) further contrasted her theory of causality with one proposed by Eldredge (1979) and Eldredge and Cracraft (1980), in which the effects of organismic stenotopy and eurytopy were seen primarily in terms of their effects on probability of extinction. In proposing that stenotopic species show higher intrinsic probabilities for speciation, Vrba (1980) confronted the difficulty that the concept of stenotopy pertains, originally and most clearly, to the economic adaptations (niche exploitation parameters) of organisms, rather than to aspects of their SMRS. If SMRSs were simply, and solely, reflections of adaptive change in economic adaptative properties of organisms, there would be no difficulty in this line of thought. But for economic adaptive specialization to be seen to affect directly the reproductive adaptations (SMRS) that are involved in speciation, a close connection between (economic) stenotopy and an equivalent version of "reproductive stenotopy" would have to be posited. Such, in fact, is precisely what Vrba (1980) invokes. Yet there is little evidence that SMRSs can be described as relatively narrow or broad, or that economic adaptations, describable in terms of relative width, are correlated with the SMRS attributes of organisms. We have already reviewed (Chap. 4) the evidence that strongly suggests that SMRS and economic adaptive features do not covary appreciably either within or among species. Indeed, if there is causal influence between the two categories of phenotypic properties, it is more likely that SMRS differentiation influences the accumulation of economic adaptive differentiation, as seems to be the case reported by Ryan and Wilczynski (1988) in cricket frogs.

The model in Chap. 4 remains the more generally compelling: SMRS disruption is hypothesized to be about equally probable in all species. On the one hand, eurytopes, tending to be rather far flung and often disjunct in their distributions, might be geographically disrupted (i.e., form geographic isolates) rather readily. On the other hand, stenotopes, with narrower distributions, might be as readily prone to patchy distributions given even slight alterations of the distributions of suitable habitats. The question seems much more a matter of what is to be expected to happen as a consequence of such enforced geographic isolation. If we allow, for the sake of argument, roughly equal probability of SMRS disruption among species that are economic eurytopes and stenotopes, is there any other causal effect arising from eurytopy and stenotopy that might lead to apparent discrepancies in speciation rates?

As argued in Chap. 4, we would expect a priori that new species that are ecologically somewhat distinct would have a greater chance for survival than species ecologically very similar to the parental species. Though early statements of this argument (e.g., Eldredge, 1979) relied rather heavily on ecological competition theory, it is really a matter of simple swamping. To gain an ecological foothold (for reasons already explored in Chap. 4), it seems plausible to assume that ecologically differentiated (derived) descendant species stand a better chance of persisting than descendants that lack significant differences from parental species.

The patterns of distribution of generalized vs. specialized species (i.e., among African cichlids and antelopes) show that closely related stenotopic species are much more likely to live sympatrically than are closely related eurytopic species. The reason, at least in general, does seem to reflect competition: generalists (eurytopes) have less to distinguish niche types than do stenotopes. Stenotopes, already specialized, seem to show a greater tendency for further economic specialization than do eurytopes. Descendant eurytopic species, on the other hand, tend to be eurytopes like the parental species—and therefore far less different from the parental species than stenotope parental and descendant species tend to be. Newly formed eurytopic species, already with a reduced probability of living sympatrically with other, closely related eurytopes, seem to have a lower initial probability of survival. Thus speciation rates are biased, even if there is an equal initial probability of SMRS disruption within eurytopes and stenotopes.

Despite the differences in theoretical arguments over the causal pathways that link niche breadth and speciation rate, biologists have in general agreed for decades that, once established, eurytopic species—which tend to be more widespread and occupy a greater variety of habitats than do stenotopes—are intrinsically more "extinction-resistant" than stenotopes. Economic specialization, in other words, increases the likelihood of extinction; and eurytopic species, indeed, do tend to display characteristically longer stratigraphic ranges than do stenotopes (see Vrba's data on the Alcelaphini vs. Aepycerotini).

Note that, regardless of precisely how considerations of niche breadth are held to affect speciation rates, both Vrba's (1980) and Eldredge's (1979; Eldredge and Cracraft, 1980) models call for the effect of organismic economic adaptations on species diversity; both look at macroevolutionary patterns, such as trends, as an interplay of (successful) speciation and extinction. In the case of trends, both see speciation acting as a ratchetlike mechanism, in which SMRS disruption conserves economic adaptive change, injecting it into the phylogenetic stream.

Species Sorting: A Final Word

The original problem that prompted the development of the species-selection literature was the need to find a deterministic cause of apparent directional change of *organismic phenotypic properties* within the context of a predominantly punctuated pattern within and among species: How could trends arise if selection favors stability of phenotypic properties for long periods of time within species? The earlier discussions spoke of species selection based on sorting (largely extinction) of species that differ in terms of the frequency distributions of the particular characters forming the trend. Because such models always focused on organismic rather than species-level properties, the term "species selection" as originally used was something of a misnomer.

Later discussions, which included origins as well as terminations of species, and which focused on emergent properties of species, brought the models closer to true selection (i.e., as a species-level analogue of natural selection) but got rather far removed from the original problem. Even the effect hypothesis (and other attempts to relate niche-breadth theory to speciation and species-extinction rates), which restored the search for species-sorting causes to the level of the organismic phenotypes, remains incompletely linked with that original problem, because the aspects of organismic phenotype pertaining to niche breadth may well *not* be those features that are observed to constitute the trend.

Thus there are two possibilities: Either species are "sorted" *because* their component organisms differ with respect to the very characters that form the trend, or the "trend" falls out strictly as a side effect of differential rates of speciation and/or extinction caused by wholly different suites of organismic characteristics. If, to these possibilities, we add the possibility of hitchhiking of organismic phenotypic characters as a side effect of "true" species selection (i.e., on species-level, emergent properties), the situation becomes even more complex.

No matter how complex the theory may seem at the moment, though, one thing is clear: Macroevolutionary theory has recently occasioned renewed interest in those biological factors that influence (if not entirely govern) rates of speciation and species extinction. These issues have not been historically well integrated with mainstream evolutionary theory—especially that aspect, the *central* aspect, that addressed patterns and underlying causes of (adaptive) anatomical change. We now pursue these issues even further in conjunction with systematics and evolutionary patterns within higher taxa.

Notes to Chapter 5

1. Because geographic boundaries are often difficult to pinpoint precisely, and because of the constant flux of composition of organisms within such local systems, many ecologists deny that ecosystems are "real entities." Other ecologists, more impressed with regularity and stability in many such systems, discount the fuzziness of boundaries (which may arise, in any case, from difficulties in the scale of human perception) and the changeable composition of such systems, choosing instead to see ecosystems as real systems, even "entities," nested, as parts, into larger systems. The debate over the reality of such systems is similar to that (Chap. 4) over the reality of species and monophyletic taxa.

2. While the majority of systematists favor recognition of the chimpanzee as the closest phylogenetic relative of *H. sapiens* among the living great apes, Schwartz (1987) has argued that orangs and humans share evolutionary novelties (synapomorphies—Chap. 6) (especially in aspects of female reproductive biology) that indicate that orangs are our closest living relative.

3. There is in fact an extensive literature on interspecific interactions, such as the notion of *character displacement* (Brown and Wilson, 1956) in evolutionary theory, and the general subject of interspecific competition in ecology. It is to be stressed at this juncture that species as wholes do not participate in interspecific competition—rather, it is individual sympatric organisms (or, at most, two different sympatric avatars) that do the competing. Competition, if it occurs at all, takes place in the context of overlapping niche characteristics of two or more avatars; entire species can only compete if one or both are reduced to the composition of a single deme–avatar.

4. I am grateful to L. Salles for convincing me (in personal conversation) that the SMRS can rationally be viewed as a species-level property.

5. For example, Fryer and Iles (1969) on African cichlid fishes; Novacek (1984) on elephant shrews; Fisher (1984) on xiphosuran arthropods; and Delson and Rosenberger (1984) on various anthropoid primates.

6. Because Vrba and other systematists can use horn morphology to assess number of species based on SMRS, the possibility of circularity is avoided in this instance. In other words, if species are recognized strictly on the basis of anatomical diversity (pertaining to economic adaptations), there is no simple way of telling whether high "speciation" rates are simply an artifact of high rates of adaptive anatomical transformation (the usual assumption in evolutionary biology), or whether indeed high speciation rates themselves constitute an actual cause of relatively high rates of anatomical change.

6

Macroevolutionary Patterns I: Genealogical Systems

The concept that there are actually two sets of organismic adaptations has already emerged as a major theme in the present discussion of macroevolutionary theory. That the economic and reproductive adaptations of organisms arise through natural and sexual selection, respectively, is a matter of Darwin's original definitions. Most crucial, perhaps, is the natural selection vector: relative economic success among conspecifics in a local population is reflected, statistically, in relative reproductive success. This is the core of the evolutionary connection between the economic and genealogical systems to which all organisms belong.

That the two classes of behavior lead to organisms' being parts of two different systems also began to emerge in the preceding chapter, when we considered the nature of species and their role in the evolutionary process. Thus, reproductive adaptations lead to organisms' being parts of demes, which are in turn parts of species; species themselves are parts of monophyletic taxa. On the other hand, the economic activities of organisms lead to their association into avatars, which are local populations of conspecifics that form the parts of local ecosystems; local ecosystems, in turn, are parts of more regional ecological systems.

From an explicitly macroevolutionary point of view, it is important to recall that most adaptations of historical concern in evolutionary theory have been of the economic kind. As functional properties, such features lead to organisms' being parts of economic systems. Yet the *histories* of such adaptations are most commonly seen as aspects of the genealogical history of life. On the one hand, this is only natural: just as organisms within single species tend to resemble each other more closely than they do organisms of other species (certainly including their economic adaptations), so members of species within higher taxa bear closer overall resemblance, especially in organismic economic adaptations, than they share with species of other higher taxa. Hence Dobzhansky's point that members of the cat family (Felidae) bear a certain adaptive resemblance to one another, as do members of the dog family (Canidae); yet canids and felids share a resemblance (with each other, and with some other families, such as bears, Ursidae) not shared with families outside the mammalian order Carnivora. There seems to be every reason to view taxa (species and higher, monophyletic taxa) as historical storehouses of genetically based information on the economic (as well as reproductive) adaptations of organisms. The information on economic adaptations is maintained (and changed) through natural selection and transmitted through the reproductive activities of organisms and the speciation process. Those reproductive activities lead to the formation of species, and species (through speciation) form higher taxa. Taxa are thus storehouses of genetically based information on adaptation.

Yet, on the other hand, the functional vs. historical aspect of economic adaptations has led to some conceptual quagmires in evolutionary theory. Thus, Dobzhansky (1951, p. 9) was right when he pointed to the families of resemblance of economic adaptation hierarchically arrayed in monophyletic taxa; but he was clearly wrong in attributing to species the *functional* characteristic of active utilization of such properties, as he did when he said that species have *niches*. The error was compounded when monophyletic taxa were said to occupy "adaptive ranges,"—additive, phylogenetically "adjacent" niches that sum up to an entire region of peaks in an adaptive landscape. Nor has Dobzhansky been the only prominent biologist to adopt this imagery that sees monophyletic taxa as parts of economic systems.

Thus the ongoing functioning of economic adaptations—forming as it does the complex ecological systems that are the subject matter of ecology—is not to be confused with the historical conservation and modification of those adaptations, which form the subject matter of evolution. But, clearly history and current function are intricately related, as the paradigm of natural selection perhaps most clearly shows. No consideration of evolution can be complete without a careful consideration of the structure and function of moment-by-moment existing economic systems. Conversely, no consideration of ecology can be complete without a consideration of source of the genetically based information that supplies the players, the organisms, to the economic arena. Thus, the final chapters of this book on the macroevolutionary aspects of the origin, maintainance, and modification of (predominantly economic) adaptations will deal first with macroevolutionary aspects of the genealogical hierarchy (this chapter), followed by a consideration of aspects of the economic hierarchy of particular macroevolutionary significance (Chap. 7), including a final discussion which considers the causal interactions between the two systems that result, in part, in macroevolution.

The Genealogical Hierarchy

The genealogical system, or *hierarchy*, is, of course, the traditional focus of evolutionary biology. The system is a hierarchy because larger-scale entities contain, as component parts, smaller-scale entities. There is a series of categories, each corresponding to individual entities (particular instances) as specific examples. For example, the category "species" contains millions of particular exemplars in the modern biota (up to 40 million, according to some recent estimates); one particular species is *Homo sapiens*. The genealogical hierarchy is summarized in Table 6.1.

The genealogical hierarchy derives as a functional entity from the "moremaking" activities of biological entities. Genes make more of themselves (replicate), a process intricately tied up with cell division. In single-celled organisms, cell division is synonymous with *reproduction*. In multicellular organisms, cell division and mitotic replication serve to make more cells of the same type, a form of reproduction, to be sure, but an aspect co-opted for the ongoing maintenance of the organismic soma. As Weismann pointed out, somatic cell division and genetic replication have no effect on those cells that take part in *organismic* reproduction:[1] it is the cells of the germ line in multicellular organisms that produce the gametes that are used in reproduction. Thus it is the germ line that is of special significance to evolutionists.

Organisms reproduce utilizing one of the available modes of cellular

TABLE 6.1   The Genealogical and Ecological
Hierarchies

Genealogical hierarchy	Ecological hierarchy
Monophyletic taxa	Biosphere
Species	Ecosystems
Demes	Avatars
Organisms	Organisms
Germ line*	Soma†

*Composed of hierarchically nested chromosomes, genes, codons, and base pairs.
†Composed of hierarchically nested organ systems, organs, tissues, cells, and proteins.
SOURCE: From Eldredge (1986), Table 1, p. 356.

division and underlying genetic replication. Thus the general mode of this biological activity is not *replication,* but simply *moremaking.* Organisms reproduce (make more of themselves) either asexually or sexually. Further, as we have seen, it is the ongoing reproductive activities of organisms that keep demes (or species) going. Sexual selection leads to stasis and occasional change in SMRSs, the basis of species maintenance and of the origin of new reproductive communities from old: speciation. Thus, as an aspect of sexual selection modifying the reproductive adaptations of organisms, species make more of themselves; speciation is the process of species' making more entities of like kind. We call strings of two or more species related by ancestry and descent *monophyletic taxa.* Because there are no larger-scale reproductive behaviors associated with such taxa of two or more species, monophyletic taxa do not "make more entities of like kind." There is no reproduction of entities of like kind above the level of species, though the literature on macroevolution is fraught with references to the derivation of one higher taxon from another, as when, for example, mammals and birds are conventionally said to be (separately) derived from "reptiles."

The genealogical hierarchy is similar to, but not to be confused with, the Linnaean hierarchy. Like the genealogical hierarchy, the Linnaean hierarchy consists of a linear list of categories; kingdom, phylum, class, order, family, genus, and species, with numerous intermediate rankings, are the category names. Each rank corresponds to numerous particular taxa: kingdom Metazoa, phylum Chordata, class Mammalia, order Primates, family Hominidae, genus *Homo,* species *Homo sapiens.* Moreover, the higher taxa are composed of taxa of lower rank: the genus *Homo,* for example, contains two other species (the extinct *H. erectus* and *H. habilis*) in addition to our own species, *H. sapiens.*

There are two fundamental reasons why the Linnaean hierarchy and the genealogical hierarchy are not the same. We have already encountered the first, and most important, reason: Because taxa of rank higher than species do not "make more of themselves," the functional, reproductive process—by which lower-level entities reproduce to make more entities of like kind to form the next higher level entity of the genealogical hierarchy—is simply absent in the Linnaean hierarchy above the level of species.

Nor is the ability of species to speciate a relevant aspect of the Linnaean hierarchy. Herein lies the germ of the second major difference between these two closely similar hierarchical systems. And there is both irony and an obvious source of confusion arising from the fact that *the Linnaean hierarchy, at least in its conceptualization as followed here, is itself a genealogical system.* The Linnaean system is genealogical in that it represents an attempt to name as taxa actual branches on the phylogenetic "tree" of life. These branches (*clades*) are defined and recognized (hence named) by the recognition of the distribution of shared derived evolutionary novelties—*synapomorphies*. As Platnick and Cameron (1977) first showed, the use of shared evolutionary novelties (morphological change injected into the phylogenetic system) is precisely the same technique as the protocol used in historical linguistics and other fields to analyze genealogical pedigrees, the actual course of ancestry and descent within any system.

Not all the branches that arise can be recognized and named. For one thing, systematists and paleontologists will never experience all taxa that have ever existed. Indeed, as Raup (1986) has stressed, most species that have ever lived have already become extinct; and most have left no trace in the fossil record. The higher up the Linnaean hierarchy one goes, the greater the chance that some species, at least, from each of the higher taxa has been discovered, analyzed, and named. Thus, at the level of phylum and kingdom, sampling should be relatively more complete than at the lower taxonomic levels.

But there is another reason why not all branches on the phylogenetic tree are named: We may have sampled some but not named them because they have lacked clear-cut, readily analyzed evolutionary novelties. We simply cannot *see* all the many branches on the historical tree of life. The practical consequences of this situation are clear: *Taxic arrangement within the Linnaean hierarchy is isomorphic with the distribution of evolutionary novelties in the phylogenetic system.* Thus deductions about the genealogical history of life rely completely on the ability of systematists to analyze the distribution of evolutionary novelties, which are phenotypic attributes of organisms. And most of *these*, of course, are economic adaptations.

Thus the Linnaean hierarchy of taxa, because of the way that taxa are defined, recognized, and named, corresponds exactly to the history of the modification of organismic phenotypes that has been shaped by the evolutionary process. As Darwin pointed out, descent with modification (with a form of branching process thrown in) automatically yields a pattern of nested resemblances linking up all forms of life. The Linnaean system recognizes this fact and takes it as its operational base. Confusion ensues when we compare the genealogical hierarchy with the Linnaean hierarchy—because both are "genealogical." One works from the bottom up: ongoing reproduction (moremaking) of lower-level entities creates the next higher entity in the genealogical hierarchy; the highest rung is reached when reproduction can no longer be seen to be a function of a particular class of entity, in this case, monophyletic taxa of rank higher than species. The other (the Linnaean system), in contrast, works from the top down, in the sense that we examine nested sets of synapomorphies to trace genealogy. It is not a question of function of entities, but of the distribution of organismic phenotypic properties (reviewed briefly below); thus the Linnaean system takes up where the genealogical system leaves off, in that the Linnaean system looks for structure within the catch-all category (i.e., of the genealogical hierarchy) of *monophyletic taxa*.

The two systems do seem to collide, however, at the level of species. In particular, the biological species concept (or, in the context of this present discussion *only*, the similar definition of species given by Paterson, e.g., 1985) seems to violate the strict "genealogical" construal of the Linnaean system, for the simple reason that biological species are often differentiated into (largely allopatric) variant subtaxa, reflecting, again, the distribution of phenotypic adaptive variation. Strict *cladists*, (systematists who take a purely genealogical view of the phylogenetic system; see below) insist that the use of synapomorphies to define genealogically pure taxa should extend down into the species level (see, e.g., Cracraft, 1987; Mishler and Brandon, 1987). Use of a "reproductive criterion" to define and recognize species would otherwise miss the fact that some parts of ancestral species, as judged from the distribution of shared phenotypic properties, *may be more closely related to a descendant species than they are to other parts of the supposed ancestral species.*

Thus, at the level of species, distribution of (largely economic) adaptations can often be at variance with the distribution of shared functional reproductive adaptations. This is actually no great surprise, given the independence in patterns of distribution and variation of reproductive and economic adaptations already encountered in this book. Problems of species definition arise only when economic adaptive differentiation has occurred on a finer scale than reproductive (SMRS) differentiation. Such a situation is most common in plants, in which morphologically well-differentiated "species" commonly hybridize. (For just this reason, botanists have been notoriously skeptical of the BSC.) To be consistent with the genealogical scheme (based on the distribution of all adaptations within a phylogenetic system[2]), some systematists insist that species not be defined and recognized according to reproductive criteria, or, more precisely, *solely* according to reproductive criteria. In their view, a single species must not include clearly differentiated subtaxa that display a pattern of genealogical interrelatedness among themselves. In contrast, as we have seen in detail in preceding chapters, from an evolutionary perspective, to be consistent with a functional moremaking scheme which seems to make sense from the lowest genetic levels on up through species and higher taxa, species must be defined and recognized, as much as is possible, on the criterion of reproductive community. What is the resolution of this apparent conflict?

In a very real sense, the conflict is simply the most recent manifestation of a deep-seated and long-standing dilemma in the conceptualization of the nature of species. When Dobzhansky (1937a) and Mayr (1942) managed to establish the primacy of a *reproductive community* concept of species, they did so at the expense of the long-established view that species are collections of anatomically similar organisms. The Linnaean system, in modern systematics, is preeminently genealogical: taxa are united by descent from a common ancestor. Because species is a traditional taxon category (i.e., like genus, family, etc.), it is a logical conclusion in many systematists' minds to require strict unity of descent for species just as for genera and higher taxa. Thus the two criteria *legitimately* lead to two different conceptualizations of species, both quite "natural"—see Donoghue (1985), who makes just this point and discusses these issues in detail. Neither, in other words, is superior to the other; neither is a "better" description of nature. The conflict that arises when purely genealogical (cladistic) considerations delimit "species" different in composition from those defined by SMRS distributions reflects a real lack of congruence in nature and is not to be passed off merely as an artifact of different ways of thinking about species. The "solution," then, to this conflict must entail recognition that there are two slightly different sets of entities that have been called "species." The reproductive (SMRS-defined) sort of unit came to biology later than the *species as taxon* notion; the BSC (and its SMRS replacement) became important only with the advent of the modern synthesis. Perhaps, then, the BSC really requires a new name. The term "species" is strongly established for both usages, however, and will continue to be used in the *reproductive community* sense throughout the remainder of this book.

Genealogically "Pure" Taxa and Macroevolution

Darwin (1859) was able to show, convincingly, why there is a nested pattern of resemblance linking up all members of the Recent biota. For at least 100 years prior to the publication of Darwin's (1859) *On the Origin of Species,* systematists (among whom Linnaeus is simply the most famous) had begun to take cognizance of the apparent structure inherent in the biological realm and to reflect that structure in "natural" classifications. Darwin's contribution to systematics was simply to show that such a pattern of nested resemblance is a necessary consequence of *descent with modification.* Put the other way around, the nested structure of the biotic realm emerges as the simplest, and strongest, prediction of what biologists *must* observe if the general notion of evolution is true.

Though aspects of the *genealogical* and *Linnaean* hierarchies clash to the point where we must see them as two related, but different, hierarchical systems, we have also already seen that both are genealogical: one (the genealogical hierarchy proper) arises out of the reproductive activities of organisms and so is quintessentially genealogical by its very nature. The Linnaean hierarchy, isomorphic with the complexly nested distribution of homologous features, is also intrinsically "genealogical," because homologous structures are transmitted in ancestry and descent in either conserved or further modified form. It should be obvious that higher taxa delineated strictly on "pure" genealogical grounds are relevant to an understanding of evolutionary process. Apparent exceptions to this generalization (as in the case of grades) involve convergence and parallelism of organismic phenotypic attributes—adaptations. This is an interesting and valid subject of evolutionary investigation *that does not require that taxa be recognized and named on patently nongenealogical criteria* to be pursued (see below for more on grades, convergence, parallelism, and nongenealogically pure taxa).

It follows that systematists take as their fundamental task the delineation of "genealogically pure" taxa. Nor is this a recent innovation: as Nelson (e.g., 1970) has pointed out, systematists even before Darwin and continuing to the present seek "natural groups," and eliminate "nonnatural" taxa that have been constructed on faulty criteria. That whales are not fish is an old (pre-Darwinian) conclusion. That large taxa such as Invertebrata are defined strictly on the absence of features that define a supposedly coordinate taxon (Vertebrata) is easily seen as an expression of ignorance. Some "invertebrates" simply must be more closely related to the vertebrates than are others, and it is the job of systematists to recognize that vertebrates are simply one group of deuterstomous, enterocoelous metazoans.

Because smaller taxa are nested within larger taxa, systematists must elucidate the genealogical relationships among a series of (already analyzed) taxa to arrive at the composition of larger-scale taxa. The methodological rules for genealogically based systematics research have, in recent years, undergone close scrutiny (see Eldredge and Cracraft, 1980; Wiley, 1981; Nelson and Platnick, 1981; Schoch, 1986). The basis of *phylogenetic systematics* (also known generally as *cladistics*) is Hennig (1950, translated into English in revised form in 1966).

The core idea of genealogically based systematics is simple: Modifications (of organismic phenotypic properties) are inherited in the same, or in further modified form, by descendants. These *evolutionary novelties* (or *synapomorphies*) are homologous structures shared by the ancestral species (in which the novelty first appears) and all its descendants. Synapomorphies (or shared derived features) serve simply as markers to recognize genealogically pure lines of descent.

Note that, once introduced, an evolutionary novelty unites an ancestral species with all its descendants, but cannot convey any further information about the genealogical structure among the descendant species. A synapomorphy that defines a taxon at one level becomes automatically a *symplesiomorphy* (shared primitive feature) when comparisons among included (descendant) taxa are made. Hair (derived over the more general amniote feature "epidermal scales") serves as a synapomorphy to delineate all Mammalia; simple presence of hair among various species of dogs (Canidae) is a primitive feature, containing no information on how various species of dogs might be interrelated. Such structure must be found in other characters, or in subsets of the general feature "hair," such as color, texture, bodily distribution, cytology, etc., of canid hair.

All phenotypic attributes of organisms have had a history. That is to say, all such features appeared at some time in phylogenetic history. This means that all features have a finite distribution in the biota. Some features are ubiquitous within all life: RNA is such a feature. Others are only slightly less generally distributed: the 9 + 2 internal structure of flagellae and cilia, uniting all Eukaryota, is an example of such a widely distributed morphological feature (Margulis, 1974). It is because the depth (in phylogenetic time) at which a novel feature is introduced is mirrored in the breadth of its distribution among different "kinds" of organisms that systematists rightly point out that a detailed fossil record (however desirable) is *not* a prerequisite for a theory of the phylogenetic relationships among living organisms, and hence for the formulation of a phylogenetic classification of living organisms.

Thus systematists must find that point in the phylogenetic history of a group at which a particular character was introduced; correctly identified, the character is a synapomorphy for the delineation of a group. This amounts to a mapping exercise: we may overestimate or underestimate the distribution of a character. There are several sources of error. The character might be present, but in such modified form that it is missed. Or we might take two similar phenotypic characters as the "same" (i.e., derived from the same condition in a common ancestor, thus *homologous*) when in fact the characters are *homoplastic*, i.e., not homologies but independently evolved and confusingly similar characters that lead to inappropriately defined, nonphylogenetically "pure" taxa. In general, the two kinds of error in systematics are (1) mistaking the true distribution of a phenotypic feature or (2) incorrectly taking two characters to be homologous when they have had separate phylogenetic histories.

Techniques of character analysis are reviewed in many different sources (see the list of general references on cladistics above). Briefly considered, there are two approaches in general use, and these, really, are aspects of the same overall method of searching for the actual distribution of characters. The first is simply to search for patterns of similarity within a data set. (The second method, study of ontogenetic transformation, is discussed below.)

All problems in systematics involve a comparison of organisms, whether all are from a single population or (more commonly) samples from different populations (in which the question might be: How many species are present in the sample?). Even more typical of modern systematics research is the investigation of the relationship among various taxa already defined and recognized (a number of species within a genus, for example), in which case the question is: What is the structure of relationships among members of the genus, hence, what is the actual genealogical composition of the genus? As another example, there may be a number of families, provisionally accepted as "genealogically pure" (*monophyletic*), in which case the question is: What are the relationships among these families?

Whatever the nature of the sample, and of the particular taxonomic level in question, the actual *form* of the problem is the same in all cases. In every analysis, there will be some aspects of organismic phenotypes which will appear not to vary from sample to sample; other features will vary to the extent that no two organisms, or any two taxa being compared, will be alike. It is the intermediate situation—in which characters seem to be shared by two or more, but not all, samples under study—that information about the structure of relationships among the taxa will be found.

There are several sources of error in evaluating the patterns of similarity among samples that emerge from those sets of phenotypic features that vary within the sample set. Any particular shared character may, of course, represent a derived evolutionary novelty, inherited from a common ancestor, and not shared with any other sample. Alternatively, the features might be homoplastic; or they may be symplesiomorphic. How can a systematist determine what the resemblances mean?

The most general approach is simply to accept, at the outset, a provisional hypothesis of relationship between the group under study and its next closest phylogenetic relative. For example, suppose the problem is to assess the relationships among the great apes and mankind (family Hominidae). Most systematists consider Old World monkeys to be the closest relatives of the hominids; they are conventionally classified together as Catarrhini. The method of *out-group* comparison is simply to examine members inside the supposed nearest relatives to see if the character in question occurs there as well: if so, it is judged to be plesiomorphic. For example, we might propose that presence of a thick coat of body hair unites all great apes into a distinct taxon—separate only from *Homo sapiens*. Consideration of Old World monkeys, though, shows hair coats to be primitive for all catarrhines (indeed, it is primitive for all mammals) and thus valueless for defining a taxon within Hominidae; in this case, it is the comparative hairlessness of humans that is derived and serves in part to define a distinctly human lineage.

The second method for assessing character distribution is the study of ontogenetic transformation of morphological features. Here, the relation between ontogeny and phylogeny is strictly analytic: study of the transformation of phenotypic features in ontogeny reveals aspects of character distribution that may not be evident from comparison strictly of adult states. Vertebrate gill slits are the classic example. Absent in the adults of amniotes and most living amphibians as gill slits (but present as highly derived structures, such as eustachian tubes in mammals), pharyngeal pockets and slits are familiar features of amniote embryos. Pharyngeal slits emerge clearly as a vertebrate synapomorphy and as a primitive feature among all living vertebrates; thus "presence of gill slits" cannot be used as a feature to unite a taxon "all fish." (However, presence of gill slits in the adult condition is not thereby demonstrably to be considered primitive in all cases; though adult gill slits are certainly primitive for vertebrates, the axolotl (a neotenic salamander) secondarily retains gills as an adult as a derived condition). Thus ontogenetic data, in conjunction with out-group comparisons, form the basis of the mapping exercise that lies at the heart of phylogenetic analysis.

Ontogenetic data contain a vector of directionality of transformation missing in the static comparison of morphologies among a series of organisms. The level at which a novelty is introduced phylogenetically is itself an issue of directionality: what is derived at one, remote level becomes primitive for later members of a lineage. Phylogenetic transformation always works on the morphology available at the moment. Thus ontogenetic data may provide an independent and (some would say) relatively direct means of inference of what form of a character is the more primitive within a series of homologous characters. Because the ontogenetic process bears a complex relation to the phylogenetic process (considered immediately below), and specifically because the order of ontogenetic events is known not always to mirror the order of phylogenetic transformation, ontogenetic data (even when available in detail) is no panacea to problems in phylogenetic reconstruction. But the observation, by embryologists, that elements of the embryonic skull and lower jaw become incorporated into the middle ear as incus and stapes bones provided the solid evidence for the derivation of these bones from the quadrate and articular bones of therapsid "reptiles." Paleontological data reveal that some therapsids had a double articulation, and further show a spectrum that can be interpreted as a switch from a quadrate-articular to an exclusively dentary-squamosal joint in mammals. But the inference is less certain, based on paleontological data alone, that the quadrate and articular actually become the incus and malleus of the mammalian middle ear.

Paleontological data, of course, do present their own directional vector: fossils come from distinct stratigraphic horizons which are naturally ordered in an older-to-younger fashion. Moreover, the vector of directionality here is precisely the same as the temporal matrix of phylogenetic change. Thus, with due caution because of the rather obvious incompleteness of the fossil record—well-analyzed, incidentally, by Darwin (1859) in his Chap. 9—many paleontologists have concluded that the fossil record is the very best source of data for phylogeny reconstruction. However, the vastly superior information of organismic attributes afforded by Recent organisms is obvious and has led some paleontologists (e.g., Patterson, 1977) to suggest that phylogenetic systems be based purely on living organisms, with such fossils as might be available for a group simply incorporated into the phylogenetic scheme derived from comparative (including ontogenetic) analysis of phenotypes of extant organisms. Utter reliance on the stratigraphic sequence of fossils to determine what states are primitive and what are derived is naive. The stratigraphic sequence *is* a valid source of inference (Fortey and Jefferies, 1982; Eldredge and Novacek, 1985), particularly at the species level, and especially when taken in conjunction with ontogenetic and out-group comparison data.

In any case, nearly all detailed cladistic studies performed so far have revealed extensive conflicts in evident distributions of synapomorphies—hence conflicting assessments of phylogenetic relationships, hence composition of taxa. Because we must assume a single phylogenetic history, conflicts automatically imply analytic error. Either symplesiomorphies have been taken for synapomorphies (in which case we have incorrectly delineated a group on the basis of shared retention of primitive features and have excluded members that should belong in that group); this is the case if we define a great-ape group (e.g., "Pongidae" of many classifications) and do not include *H. sapiens*. Or we may have taken synapomorphies as symplesiomorphies (i.e., failed to recognize phylogenetic structure where it in fact exists). Or we may simply have taken homoplastic characters as homologies, a relatively common occurrence in the history of systematics.

Before examining the consequences for evolutionary theory of defining monophyletic (genealogically pure) and nonmonophyletic higher taxa, a brief discussion on the process aspects of ontogeny—specifically, how ontogeny is related to the phylogenetic transformation of phenotypic properties—is relevant.

Heterochrony and the Two Classes of Phenotypic Adaptation

Van Valen (1976) once defined evolution as the "control of development by ecology." To get adaptive change in evolution, it is obviously necessary to modify the pathways of ontogeny, and though Van Valen's aphorism glosses over the entire issue of selection acting on heritable variation in adaptive phenotypic properties, there *is* truth in his statement. Many theorists have seen processes of change in the timing and expression of morphogenesis as an aspect of the evolutionary process itself: for example, factors intrinsic to the developmental process are often seen as promoters or triggers of modification of developmental pathways, allowing some transformations to occur, while inhibiting or preventing altogether the appearance of other possible morphologies. Indeed, the basis of some theories of macroevolution—e.g., those of the geneticist Richard Goldschmidt (1940)—look to disruptions of ontogeny through "macromutations" as a major source of phenotypic transformation in evolution.

Though at first glance theories that explain phenotypic transformation with reference to internalist, developmental processes are irrelevant to an understanding of adaptation, the two approaches do intersect if ontogenetic modification is viewed simply as an aspect of the origin of variation, which natural selection can either accept or reject. Most major disruptions of ontogeny are not viable, which amounts simply to the crudest form of selection. Nonetheless, because this book focuses largely on the large-scale, biotic context of adaptive change (where the causation underlying organic design in nature is seen to arise from the environment as the origin of selective "forces" working on heritable variation), we will not deal further with supposed processes of development sometimes said to be involved in macroevolution.

Yet, whether regarded as process, or simply as pattern, changes in the (relative) timing of the development of phenotypic structures in ontogeny are relevant to the present discussion because, once again, the relation between the two classes of phenotypic properties—economic, or somatic, features vs. reproductive features—appears to be crucial to an understanding of the phenomenon.[3]

Heterochrony is the general term used in evolutionary biology to embrace the change in relative timing of ontogenetic events that underlie phylogenetic transformation of morphological features (see Gould, 1977). In general, a feature might begin to develop either earlier or later in the ontogeny of the descendant than it does in the ancestral taxon. Gould (1977), Alberch et al. (1979), and others have discussed the possible ways to establish standard points of reference against which relatively *earlier* and *later* might be established. It is the timing of the beginning of development of one character vs. another which is of especial interest in the present context.

Clearly, the timing of any one somatic (economic) character relative to another can, and often does, change in ontogeny. Because it is empirically true that some somatic features (generally the vast majority) remain relatively stable while a minority undergo change—a point Simpson (1944, Chap. 1) discusses thoroughly, for example—it must be true that such "general heterochrony" (changes in developmental timing between any two somatic features) occurs as a matter of course in phylogeny.

However, it is the juxtaposition of the timing of *initiation* of development of particular somatic features and the *conclusion* of development of reproductive features which has provoked the greatest attention in the heterochrony literature. Hence the basis of modern classifications of modes of heterochrony.[4] Thus, if sexual maturity is reached earlier with respect to an aspect of somatic development, the resultant pattern is (phylogenetic) *paedomorphosis*. Descendant adult organisms resemble in one or more aspects of the somatic phenotypes the juveniles of the ancestors. Paedomorphosis may occur in either of two ways: either sexual maturity itself is speeded up (*progenesis*) or development of somatic features is retarded with respect to the onset of sexual maturity (*neoteny*).

In *peramorphosis* (Alberch et al., 1979), in contrast, earlier stages of a descendant's somatic morphology resemble the adult stages of the ancestor: the ontogeny of the descendant "goes beyond" the final stages of development in the ancestor. This is the phenomenon of *recapitulation*, of which there are two forms. *Acceleration* is the peramorphic equivalent (and exact opposite) of neoteny: in acceleration, aspects of the development of the soma are speeded up, relative to the onset of reproductive maturation. *Hypermorphosis,* on the other hand, is the peramorphic equivalent (and exact opposite) of progenesis: reproductive maturity is delayed relative to the development of aspects of the somatic phenotype.

Moreover, one can readily imagine situations in which both reproductive and somatic features were speeded up—or slowed down—in concert. In practice, it is often difficult to distinguish what mode of paedomorphosis or peramorphosis has occurred. Note, too, that while it makes sense to retain the basic classification based on the difference between paedomorphosis and peramorphosis, another way to classify these heterochronic events would be to stress the dichotomy between economic and reproductive features: peramorphic and paedormophic effects arise either from (1) slowing down or speeding up the onset of reproductive maturity, with rates of development of nonreproductive features remaining unchanged from ancestor to descendant, or from (2) speeding up or slowing down the timing of development events of the soma, with the rate of sexual maturation remaining constant from ancestor to descendant. From the standpoint of classifying similar effects (i.e., peramorphosis vs. paedomorphosis), clearly the well-established system discussed by Gould (1977), Alberch et al. (1979), McNamara (1986), and others is to be preferred. From the standpoint of understanding the processes underlying such patterns (and linking them with a theme of great importance in other aspects of macroevolutionary theory), the system based on the dichotomy between economic and reproductive systems might be preferable.

That patterns of phylogenetic heterochrony are often understood to arise in changes in the relative timing of the development of economic and reproductive phenotypic features is important to the overall consideration of adaptive change in evolution primarily because it underscores the tendency for such sets of features to vary at least semi-independently. Within species, i.e., within a shared fertilization system (SMRS), there may be a great deal of economic variation (whether intra- or interpopulational), or relatively little economic differentiation. In relation to speciation, we have seen that there is an asymmetrical relation: changes in SMRS (i.e., to form new species) may or may not be accompanied by significant changes in economic adaptations; however, little in the way of economic change seems to be incorporated into phylogeny *without* SMRS change. Similarly, variation in rates of sexual maturation and of economic (somatic) development with respect to one another and to organismic age are well established in Recent populations of organisms, certainly including *H. sapiens*. That such variation can be translated into generation-by-generation change is also apparent, as in the instances of changes in age of onset of reproductive maturity in human populations. But the literature on evolutionary heterochrony seems to suggest an even greater independence between economic and reproductive systems in organisms, such that variations in rate of development of one system with respect to the other are easily, and commonly, translated into the basis of the development of morphological change in phylogeny.

Macroevolutionary Patterns Within Higher Taxa

The *new systematics* (a term, like the *modern synthesis,* coined by J. Huxley in the early 1940s) was the approach to systematics methodologically consistent with the theory of the evolutionary process of the synthesis itself. Perhaps not surprisingly, much of new systematics dealt with the recognition of polytypic species and with patterns of within-species variation. Also not surprising is the fact that it was Simpson (1945, 1961 in particular) and Mayr (1942 in part; also Mayr, Linsley, and Usinger, 1953; and Mayr, 1969) who were the major exponents of new systematics praxis; Simpson, especially, was concerned with the principles of phylogenetic reconstruction and classification of higher taxa.

Simpson (e.g., 1975) and Mayr (1974) have remained staunch opponents of Hennig's approach to phylogenetic systematics, yet each has conceded that synapomorphies are nested and that the correct analysis of the point in the phylogenetic history of a taxon at which an evolutionary novelty appears constitutes the one logical guide to the course of phylogenetic relationships within a higher taxon. Yet, Simpson and Mayr (and many others) continue to maintain that a genealogical system alone should not form the basis of a classification, either because hierarchically arrayed genealogies cannot be expressed in the Linnaean system (e.g., Mayr, 1942, p. 277—clearly an erroneous conclusion) or because elements of evolutionary information other than the purely genealogical will be left out of a classification. The subject of classification lies beyond the scope of this book; suffice it to say, debate continues to rage, with cladists (e.g., Farris, 1977) maintaining that genealogically based classifications in fact maximize the predictive power of classifications, when "predictivity" means expected distribution of additional similarities not already used as the basis of classification.

From the standpoint of evolutionary theory per se, because evolution is a quintessentially genealogical process, cladists not surprisingly maintain that only genealogically pure taxa should be the object of evolutionary analysis. Taxa originate, have histories, and eventually terminate. Prior to the widespread adoption of cladism, systematists concerned with the relationships of higher taxa of organisms generally adopted Simpson's (e.g., 1961, p. 124) definition of *monophyly* or one like it: "Monophyly is the derivation of a taxon through one or more lineages from one immediately ancestral taxon of the same or lower rank." Evolutionary systematists have routinely recognized as monophyletic many taxa that phylogenetic systematists would consider either *paraphyletic* (i.e., taxa which contain only some of the known descendants of an ancestral species) or *polyphyletic* (i.e., taxa which contain some elements not united by descent from a common ancestor).

Phylogenetic systematists recognize that there must be *genealogical structure* to any proposition that states that taxon *A* is ancestral to taxon *B:* obviously, some species within taxon *A* are more closely related to those in taxon B than others are, a fact that should be recognized in classification schemes as well as in whatever forms of evolutionary explanation are brought to bear on the evolution of higher taxa. For example, consistent with Simpson's definition of monophyly, many evolutionary systematists argue that the family Hominidae (including only the genus *Homo,* plus the extinct genus *Australopithecus*) descended from the family Pongidae (extant great apes, plus extinct relatives). But the statement "Family Pongidae is ancestral to family Hominidae" ignores the conventionally accepted hypothesis (reviewed above in another context) that species of the genus *Pan* are more closely related to *Homo* than are other members of the "Pongidae." To phylogenetic systematists, the family Pongidae does not exist (because it excludes the descendant species allocated to the genera *Australopithecus* and *Homo*). What, then, does it mean to discuss the origin of a "family" such as "Pongidae"?

We have already seen that there is *no* true theory addressed to the origin of taxa of any rank *except species*. There is no process of the origin of genera, families, orders, and so forth comparable to the speciation process, though Simpson (1944, p. 199), for example, did characterize his model of quantum evolution as "most important and distinctive at relatively high levels." Examined in detail, all such models of the origin of higher taxa are actually theories of the origin of adaptations, not of taxa per se. Simpson's (1959a) paper on the "nature and origin of supraspecific taxa" is actually a statement of the modes of origins of adaptations; it was here, for example, that he discussed the notion of *key innovations* (see Chap. 2) and the effect that such novelties might be expected to have on the evolutionary proliferation that forms *adaptive radiations*.

Thus, ironically, all systematists agree that questions pertaining to the origin of higher taxa (however those taxa are defined) boil down to modes of origin of organismic phenotypic properties—*evolutionary novelties,* or, most simply, *adaptations,* that serve as markers, or *synapomorphies,* to demarcate lineages. Monophyly (in a strict, cladistic sense) is isomorphic (i.e., the exact topological equivalent) with the distribution of synapomorphy. And synapomorphy distribution *is* the history of introduction of adaptive novelty in the phylogenetic stream. Yet, purely from the standpoint of the history of adaptations, it may make little difference if a taxon under study itself is paraphyletic; the important issue is the study of the distribution of the characters themselves. For example, any discussion of the origin of the "Pongidae" would amount to a discussion of the origin of the distinguishing phenotypic characters found within the group; a phylogenetic systematist would not recognize "Pongidae," but would address the origin of the synapomorphies for the Hominidae (i.e., extant and fossil great apes, plus *Homo* and *Australopithecus*) and would thereby confront exactly the same suite of features that an evolutionary systematist would characterize as "pongid."

Frankly polyphyletic taxa, on the other hand, would seem to constitute a case in which nonmonophyly *does* make a difference to the analysis of mode of origin of a taxon. It was fashionable, in the late 1950s and early 1960s, to recognize many traditionally accepted taxa as polyphyletic. Rather than descending from a single common ancestral species, members of such polyphyletic taxa traced separate ancestries from several different species. When the various ancestral species are sufficiently closely related to warrant inclusion in a higher taxon of rank roughly equal to that of the descendant taxon (thus actually conforming to Simpson's broad conceptualization of monophyly), the shared similarities that caused the descendant species all to be included in the descendant higher taxa were said to arise from *parallelism*—independent derivation of similar adaptations. More blatantly polyphyletic taxa were said to arise from *convergence*—in which closely similar adaptations were said to arise from nonhomologous states in disparate ancestral groups. In practice, there is no hard and fast discriminatory rule separating paralellism from convergence. The atlas-axis complex of birds and mammals, apparently independently derived from the primitive amniote ("reptile") condition, exemplifies parallelism (Schaeffer et al., 1972); the similarities between porpoises, ichthyosaurs, and sharks, on the other hand, is more obviously convergence, though no biologists in modern times, whatever their theoretical evolutionary perspective, have advocated lumping those three taxa together to form a larger taxon.

The theoretical presuppositions underlying the recognition of polyphyletic taxa are clear: the power of natural selection was generally held to be so pervasive that, given the necessary structural precursors and genetic variability, it was seen as inevitable that certain adaptive configurations would always arise. They are likely to do so at different times and places in phylogenetic history, given similar environments and similar biological starting materials. Convergence *is* an important aspect of evolution, certainly helping to illustrate the pervasive nature of adaptation as the central cause of apparent design in nature. Moreover, no one (certainly no phylogenetic systematist) would argue that it is undesirable to identify polyphyletic taxa. The difference between evolutionary and phylogenetic systematists lies in what is made of the discovery of a polyphyletic taxon: The cladist thinks that error has been revealed and hastens to realign component species into properly construed monophyletic taxa. The evolutionary systematist, on the other hand, welcomes the discovery as illustrative of evolutionary processes and is more than happy to retain such a taxon.

Acceptance of polyphyletic taxa reached a peak shortly after publication of Huxley's (1958) influential paper on *grades* and *clades* (see Chap. 2 for discussion). A *grade* is a level of shared adaptive structural complexity; if reached one time (i.e., within a single ancestral species), the adaptive configuration constitutes a synapomorphy and the resultant taxon is monophyletic. More usually, the adaptive configuration is thought to arise more than once (because of the powerful, repetitive influence of natural selection) and the taxon is nonmonophyletic. Thus, as discussed more fully in Chap. 2, Simpson (1959*b*) pronounced Mammalia to be polyphyletic, claiming that "mammals" arose many separate times (based on his analysis, largely, of fossil taxa). Instead of proposing to divide "Mammalia" so-construed into a number of monophyletic taxa, Simpson instead pointed to the virtual inevitability of the development of mammalian-type features from the "reptilian" grade. Later systematists have, apparently universally, rejected Simpson's (1959*b*) analysis, seeing all modern mammals as a monophyletic taxon that includes a number of fossil taxa provisionally allocated.

The argument that a particular taxon is polyphyletic should entail the demonstration that some of the subsidiary taxa assigned to it are in fact more closely related (i.e., genealogically) to taxa *not* included in the taxon. Such a demonstration is usually followed by the removal of the erroneously classified taxa from the larger, nonmonophyletic taxon. However, biologists intent upon recognizing polyphyletic grades generally base *their* conclusions on an entirely different style of argumentation: characters are often held to be parallelisms or convergences (rather than synapomorphies) because their manifest adaptive nature (often perceived in conjunction with functional anatomical analysis, see Chap. 2) suggests that they may, indeed in all probability *did*, arise "more than once." This is precisely the argument underlying the claim, for example, that the Arthropoda are a structural grade, polyphyletically derived from Annelida (or annelid-like ancestors), an interpretation upheld, for example, by Tiegs and Manton (1958) and a number of subsequent arthropod students. Others interested in arthropod phylogeny point out that the simplest explanation for the shared anatomical features that appear to unite Arthopoda as a monophyletic group is to imagine them having arisen but once. Many of the similarities that do appear to unite Arthropoda into a monophyletic taxon (such as aspects of the biochemistry of the exoskeleton) are perfectly reasonable putative synapomorphies and are not counterbalanced by other character distributions indicating any subsection of Arthropoda to be in fact more closely related to any other group of organisms, annelid or otherwise. Thus the argument for polyphyly is usually vague, invoking parallelism or convergence because some perceived functional value of a character suggests to a systematist that the character could easily have evolved more than once in the course of evolutionary history.

It should be added, however, that the actual functional-evolutionary analysis underlying the origin of the adaptations themselves (whether viewed as synapomorphies or parallelisms) must be evaluated on its own merits in any particular case. That polyphyletic taxa make no sense from an evolutionary point of view does not mean that similar adaptations do not arise more than once. As long as the analysis is addressed to the patterns of organismic phenotypic change (and not taken to be addressed to the origin of the taxa per se), whether the taxon is monophyletic or not is not particularly germane. What *is* germane is the frequency of parallelism vs. the single-event origin of most adaptations. Many systematists (cladists) in recent years, noting the almost inevitable occurrence of character conflict in their analyses (i.e., when more than one cladogram emerges as a possible resolution of the data), have realized that parallelism is, if anything, more common in evolutionary history than even its most ardent, grade-oriented earlier champions ever thought!

Taxa, in addition to originating, also become extinct. They do so by the extinction of component species, which is generally a matter of death of component organisms.[5] Naturally, if a taxon is polyphyletic, it will appear to survive longer if just one of the component taxa of such a nongenealogical group manages to avoid extinction. The issue of mono-, para-, and polyphyletic status of taxa has recently become a source of intense interest in macroevolution, in concert with attempts to build and analyze data bases pertaining to mass extinction. (Mass extinction is a cross-genealogical, hence ecological, issue, to which we return in the following chapter.) However, extinction is registered in the genealogical hierarchy (and measured by biologists) as the extinction of taxa. Definition of taxa, naturally, would seem to play an important role in the interpretation of any apparent patterns of differential longevity they may display.

As we have seen, macroevolutionary formulations in the synthesis, especially under Simpson's rather loose concept of monophyly, allow one higher taxon to be ancestral to another (even in the absence of any explicit process theory unique to higher taxa to explain such modes of origin). Accordingly, an ancestral taxon so conceived could be viewed as becoming extinct in two ways: (1) through "real" extinction, i.e., by extinction of all component species, or (2) by "pseudoextinction," or "extinction by transformation," in which the ancestor disappears by evolving into its descendant. Paraphyletic taxa—which omit derived, well-demarcated lineages—are in fact such "ancestral" taxa, defined as distinct units only by the lack of the derived characters of the advanced lineages. Cladists (e.g., Patterson and Smith, 1987) have expressed concern that many of the taxa (specifically, fish and echinoderm families) compiled by Sepkoski (1982) may actually be going extinct by such taxonomic artifact, amounting to pseudoextinction. However, as Van Valen (1973) points out (and because true pseudoextinction cannot occur), paraphyletic "ancestral" taxa are almost certain to live on as a collateral lineage alongside the more derived lineage (apes live alongside *H. sapiens,* at least for the moment—even if they are construed as constituting the paraphyletic family Pongidae).[6] Thus there is some merit to Sepkoski's (1987) position that extinction of such paraphyletic taxa does register species loss and thus is germane to analysis of extinction phenomena.

In addition to periods of origination and extinction, there are (usually considerable) periods of time when a monophyletic taxon is in existence; the average length is usually in rough proportion to rank. Phyla last longer than genera. It is within such taxa throughout their histories that many of the classic "macroevolutionary" patterns are found: trends (see Chap. 5); adaptive radiations; arrested evolution (the phenomenon of "living fossils,"); and the "steady state" phenomenon (Eldredge and Cracraft, 1980), in which speciation and species extinction are accompanied by little major adaptive change through time. It is important to note that while each pattern can (and should) be discussed in the context of species and higher taxa, the patterns themselves are defined and recognized as typical phylogenetic histories *of adaptive phenotypic properties of organisms.* This is the original, and still valid, conception of each of these four macroevolutionary patterns briefly to be discussed in this section.

Each of these patterns can be characterized as rising from an interplay of rates of speciation and extinction, with associated characteristic degrees, kinds, and directions of adaptive change. Eldredge and Cracraft (1980, Chap. 6; see Table 6.2) sought connections between niche width, speciation and extinction rates, and morphological change in their classification and characterization of these four basic macroevolutionary patterns. In general, such theory is in its infancy; heretofore, such patterns were almost exclusively considered a func-

TABLE 6.2 Macroevolutionary Patterns: Criteria for Recognition, Modes of Species Selection, and Predictions Concerning Component Species

Macroevolutionary pattern	Criteria							Predictions	
	Diversity pattern	Sp/ext. ratio*	Sp. rate*	Spp. sel.*	Ext. rate*	Eury./steno.*		Geog. dist.*	Apo./plesio.*
Adaptive radiation	Many closely related species arising in a short period of time	≥ 1, later, ~1	High	Disruptive	High	Mostly stenotopes; much sympatry		Narrow	Many autapomorphies; plesiomorphies relatively few
Arrested evolution	Low diversity for long periods of time	~1	Low	Neutral	Low	Eurytopes; little sympatry		Wide	Much retention of plesiomorphies; autapomorphies rare
Steady state	Moderate diversity for long periods; occasional adjustments in equilibrium value	~1	Moderate to high	Neutral or centripetal	Moderate to rapid	Mixed		Varied	Some subgroups with autapomorphies; some retention of pleisomorphies
Trends	Varied, usually low diversity	~1	Moderate to high	Directional	Moderate to rapid	Stenotopy dominant		Narrow	Clinal, progressive replacement of successively more apomorphic states

*ABBREVIATIONS: Sp./ext. ratio = ratio of speciation and extinction; sp. rate = speciation rate; spp. sel. = mode of species selection; ext. rate = extinction rate; eury./steno. = degree to which component species are eurytopic or stenotopic; geog. dist. = relative geographical distribution of component species; apo./plesio. = relative degree of apomorphy and plesiomorphy of component species.
SOURCE: From Eldredge and Cracraft (1980), Table 6.1, p. 313.

tion of rates of adaptive change, without explicit reference to speciation or species extinction (but see Bock, 1979).

Adaptive Radiations

There is little beyond the descriptive that might rightfully be called "adaptive radiation theory." Marsupial evolution in Australia affords perhaps *the* classic example; marsupials occupy a wide variety of ecological niches in Australia and Tasmania, coincidentally paralleling developments in placental mammalian evolution elsewhere, as in the Tasmanian wolf, with its resemblance to placental wolves of the northern hemisphere (not to mention its resemblance to other marsupial, but not closely related, thylacine carnivores of the Tertiary of South America).

Yet there are some recurrent elements to adaptive radiations that allow the rudiments of a causal theory to emerge. Thus, speciation and extinction rates seem to be high, especially in early phases. This implies that species are relatively stenotopic, and just as in the development of trends within stenotopic lineages (Chap. 5), synapomorphies are therefore accrued at a relatively rapid rate. As the term "radiation" implies, the overall pattern of phenotypic adaptive change is *centrifugal,* merely a descriptive characterization of the invasion of many different niches, thus the development of an array of different apomorphies (evolutionary novelties).

Thus "adaptive radiation" usually refers to *economic* adaptations. The term "radiation" suggests invasion into a variety of "empty" niches, or, more generally, the building of complex ecosystems where only simpler systems (or no systems at all, as in new environments or following mass extinctions) had formerly existed. Often biologists imply that the ecological opportunity itself triggers such radiations. However, as we reviewed in detail in Chap. 4, it is difficult to see how selective pressure for economic adaptive change itself leads to the disruption of SMRS, which is the sine qua non of the speciation process. It is likely that survival of newly formed species increases dramatically in situations in which relatively few taxa are available to establish ecosystems in general habitat settings capable of supporting taxically highly diverse systems.

Thus speciation—true speciation, involving the disruption of SMRS—is a major, if under-recognized, aspect of adaptive radiations. This is to say that changes in reproductive adaptations play an important role, in addition to the more obvious economic adaptive changes that are the central focus of this particular evolutionary pattern. But there are, in addition, adaptive radiations in which most of the change seems concentrated in the reproductive, rather than the economic, adaptive aspects of the component organismic phenotypes. For example, the great diversity of floral morphologies within the southern African family Proteaceae (accompanied, of course, with a degree of ecological diversity as well) is apparently a case in point. And although there is considerable ecological diversification (e.g., in feeding behavior) within the immense radiation of fruit flies on the Hawaian Islands (comprising some 750 species), many of the species are apparently ecologically nearly "redundant." Diversity is maintained through (at least partial) allopatry, microhabitat differences, and, of course, differences in SMRS systems. To be sure, economic differentiation can be subtle, and presumably underlies extensive coexistence of all sibling species. But the point here is that some adaptive radiations involve spectacular and obvious adaptive modifications (including the development of highly specialized economic adaptations), while other radiations are much more "modest"—yet may entail as many species. The difference is that in one instance, there is a great deal of economic change in concert with reproductive adaptive change, whereas in other instances, the same amount of SMRS change (i.e., number of species) results in far smaller amounts of economic adaptive change. The point of further research on adaptive radiations is to specify the conditions under which high speciation rate yields comparably high rates of accumulation of economic change, and when it does not.

Any contemplation of the phylogenetic relationships among a series of species constituting an adaptive radiation reveals a wealth of "substructural" detail. There are monophyletic subclades, within which there might be trends, or relatively little accumulation through time of economic adaptive change. Adaptive radiations, then, are (generally rather rapid) proliferations of species constituting a monophyletic taxon. The whole group yields the radiation, while subcomponents might themselves diversify, remain adaptively rather uniform, or develop one or more directional trends. Eldredge and Cracraft (1980) discuss the radiation (in presumably economic characteristics) within a monophyletic family of trilobites (Calmoniidae) of the southern hemisphere Siluro-Devonian. Though the entire diverse array would seem to qualify as a radiation, examination of the composition and separate histories of several sublineages (hypothesized to be monophyletic) reveals a mixture of trends, steady state (i.e., little adaptive change), and diversification. In particular, after an initial diversification, most of the diversity in later stages of the history of the Calmoniidae appears to stem from a single monophyletic subgroup derived from the initial period of diversification.

Thus there is no single, coherent pattern always to be found that constitutes the macroevolutionary pattern "adaptive radiation." Recognition that speciation is always involved, that economic change bears a complex relation to speciation, and that economic adaptive change is not always marked in the diversification of monophyletic lineages sharpens the picture a bit on adaptive radiations, as does the realization that adaptive radiations are in fact complex mosaics of other sorts of phylogenetic patterns. Adaptive radiations, as real phenomena of phylogenetic history, offer an opportunity for further empirical and theoretical investigation; they offer, as well, a challenge for a better integration of neo-Darwinian adaptive theory and the emerging theory of taxic evolution.

Arrested Evolution

Simpson (1944) recognized three discrete categories of evolutionary rates—*bradytely,* for slow rates, *horotely* for "normal" rates, and *tachytely* for high rates. Though his contention that these three classes of evolutionary rates are qualitatively distinct (i.e., not just occupying the two tails and midrange of a single curve of evolutionary rates) is dubious (Eldredge, 1984; Stanley, 1984), Simpson convincingly called the phenomenon of *arrested evolution* to theoretical attention. Simpson's interest in bradytely stemmed from the frustration that the very evidence for extremely *high* rates of morphological transformation is missing, represented by gaps in the fossil record; thus, if extremely *slow* rates could be seen as the inverse of high rates, the conditions that promote one could shed light on those that cause the other. And the data on slow-rate lines in the fossil record is often good.

Schopf (1984), Eldredge (1984), and Stanley (1984) have discussed the many variant definitions of arrested evolution (and the phenomenon of "living fossils"). In general, the pattern pertains to monophyletic taxa in which very little morphological change has accrued since the inception of the lineage. Some well-demarcated lineages are very old. Essentially anatomically modern horseshoe crabs first appear in the Upper Paleozoic; lungfish and coelacanths arose in the Devonian, and, after each underwent initial periods of adaptive differentiation (radiation), little adaptive change has accrued in either line since Carboniferous times.[7]

Though not all putative examples of arrested evolution display the following ingredients of a casual pattern, some—including horseshoe crabs (Eldredge, 1979), impalas (Vrba, 1984*b*), elephant shrews (Novacek, 1984), and other groups—display some or all of the following characteristics: low species diversity at any one point in time, long species durations, and widespread geographic distributions. In other words, as developed at greater length in Chap. 5, low-rate lineages appear to be formed of eurytopes, which, as argued earlier, tend as a rule to accrue adaptive change very slowly.

Two additional points not covered in Chap. 5 are relevant here. First of all, there is indeed a chicken-and-egg dilemma involving cause and effect in the analysis of correlation of low rates of anatomical change with low rates of speciation. As set forth in Chap. 4, if species are nothing but arbitrarily defined packages of morphological similarity, the rate of appearance of species is a direct and rather simple function of the rate of anatomical change. Thus low species diversity is a result, not a cause, of rates of evolutionary phenotypic change. In contrast, if species are reproductive communities, and if speciation is a function of the modification of fertilization systems, then low species diversity is more than likely a cause—not an effect— of low rates of morphological transformation.

Secondly, resistance to extinction of eurytopic species is not held to be the same as arrested evolution per se. Some authors (e.g., Schopf, 1984) have taken living fossils to be representatives of the *same species* living, in some instances, for hundreds of millions of years. In contrast, when the term "living fossil" is used accurately, it simply refers to low rates of anatomical change accrued over such periods of time. The species are not held literally to be the same. Rather, the resistance to extinction displayed by component species is relative (certainly not absolute!) and is causally implicated in the survival of new species in the lineage (as discussed in Chap. 5). The relevance of eurytopy to extinction is further briefly explored in the next chapter, under the discussion on mass extinctions.

Steady State

Most monophyletic taxa throughout most of their existence display little noteworthy accrual of adaptive change. Mammalian evolution since the Oligocene has produced relatively little in the way of adaptive novelty, with the possible exception of consciousness and other unusual mental attrib es of a few species of primates. Though there is even less in the way of systematic structural pattern to such phylogenetic histories than can be found in adaptive radiations, nonetheless they are absolutely characteristic of the vast majority of phylogenetic lineages known. Eldredge and Cracraft (1980) referred to such periods as *steady state* and tried to characterize the patterns in the same niche-width and rate parameters as trends, adaptive radiations, and arrested evolution.

There is little to be said about steady state, except that most of taxic macroevolution involves relatively little evolutionary activity beyond rather humdrum speciation and species extinction. Just as the vast bulk of the phylogenetic adaptive history *within* a species seems to be relative stasis, so it seems to be with many monophyletic taxa. Trilobites diversified in the Cambrian and were cut back severely several times by extinctions; by the Ordovician the last clades that were well marked by obvious and evident synapomorphies had appeared. The remaining 200 + million years of trilobite evolution were marked by the stepwise elimination of clades, and by occasional rather modest bursts of adaptive modification. The final clade of trilobites to become extinct (and the only clade to survive the Devonian and live through the last 120 million years of the Paleozoic: the Proetacea) arose in the Ordovician; and Permian species end up looking not unlike their remote Ordovician progenitors. Evolutionists have always focused on the examples of obvious, dramatic change. Most of phylogenetic history, at whatever taxonomic level, is more a matter of variations on a theme than constant and substantial phenotypic transformation.

Summary: Monophyly of Higher Taxa and Macroevolutionary Theory

Higher taxa, if they are defined and recognized by the introduction of evolutionary novelties, are actual branches of the phylogenetic "tree" of life's history. Evolutionary novelties are modifications of preexisting organismic phenotypic attributes, and thus homologies that are complexly internested according to the order of their introduction in evolutionary history. When evolutionary novelties are correctly mapped, they are synapomorphies that demarcate monophyletic taxa. Because the nested patterns of synapomorphy represent best estimates of the actual course of adaptive transformation, the genealogical system that is isomorphic with the nested pattern of synapomorphy is the logical taxic system for study of the history of adaptive change. This is seen especially clearly in the example of fish morphological evolution by Schaefer and Lauder (1986), discussed in Chap. 2.

As real entities, monophyletic taxa have beginnings, histories, and terminations. Because species are the highest-level taxon that give rise to descendant taxa, the "origin" of a higher monophyletic taxon entails nothing more than the acquisition of a particular and readily apparent (to a systematist) adaptive modification, and the transmission of that novelty to descendant species. The literature on the origin of higher taxa in general is geared to an explanation of adaptive change, not to higher taxa per se.

Polyphyletic taxa, based on nonhomologous similarities, mask the actual course of events of adaptive change. Even when such groups are understood to be polyphyletic, the actual sequence of events leading to the emergence of adaptive transformation is likely to be obscured by the inclusion of unrelated taxa within the same higher taxon. Paraphyletic taxa, on the other hand, pose less difficulty in the analysis of adaptive transformation, because paraphyletic groups omit some derived (later) sublineages: paraphyletic taxa are "defined" as those members of a larger taxon that lack further derived phenotypic attributes. The higher taxon to which the paraphyletic (ancestral) and derived taxa both belong, however, is defined on the very same set of synapomorphies (adaptations) in cladistics as the set of characters used to characterize the (paraphyletic) ancestral taxon alone in evolutionary systematics.

Extinction, on the other hand, does not coincide with a loss (by transformation) of adaptive features; rather, true extinction represents actual loss of taxa, through extinction of all component species within the higher taxon. Extinction of species, of course, amounts to loss of all constituent organisms, obviously including their adaptive features. Because of the difficulties inherent in paleontological data at the species level (only a fraction of species that have ever existed are likely ever to be sampled in the fossil record), measurements of species diversity are estimated through use of higher taxa. The higher ranked a taxon, the more species it is likely to contain, and the more likely it is that the taxon will be included in a sample. On the other hand, because many species can become extinct without the entire phylum or class to which they all belong becoming extinct, the higher ranked the taxon, the less sensitive it will be to species-level patterns of extinction. Thus there is a compromise position—taxa around the level of family seem indicated as the best choice to maximize sampling and yet also to retain sensitivity to species-level phenomena. Though thoroughly monophyletic taxa remain the ideal in compilations of extinction phenomena, it must be borne in mind that even paraphyletic families represent extinction activity at the species level (unless the only phenomenon being recorded is the pseudoextinction arising from transformation of features, already discussed above and considered highly unlikely). Polyphyletic taxa, on the other hand, can be of only marginal utility in compiling extinction data, if for no reason other than the greater probability of survival that such taxa surely have: a polyphyletic "family" may survive an extinction event, masking the extinction of a monophyletic subclade.

It is in the macroevolutionary analysis of the actual histories of taxa that the importance of monophyly is clearest. Trends, adaptive radiations, arrested evolution, and steady state are all based on perceived patterns of evolutionary stasis and change of organismic phenotypic attributes within higher taxa. Such patterns make little sense if the taxon is not genealogically coherent. The point is all the more obvious when it is realized that the genealogical structure of a taxon is based on synapomorphies, and synapomorphies *are* the history of morphological change within a taxon.

As reviewed in detail in Chap. 4, speciation is now emerging as an important causal element of adaptive change. Extinction (of species) changes the complexion of the pools of genetic information available for both the restocking of ecosystems (Chap. 7) and, in a more conventionally evolutionary sense, further evolutionary transformation.

Thus higher taxa *are* coherent pools of genetic information. It is in this sense that Dobzhansky's (1951, pp. 9–10, quoted on p. 19) imagery of species perched on peaks, with related species on adjacent peaks forming entire "ranges" on the landscape, has definite validity. But these are not "adaptive" peaks and ranges, nor are they "fitness" peaks. Each peak, rather, is simply a description of the genetic information within each species, rather like the multiple-peak picture developed originally by Wright (1931) for the description of genetic information within species.

Because monophyletic taxa are genealogical strings of species, and because species are not interactors in any direct, economic sense (Chap. 5), monophyletic taxa likewise cannot be interactors. Like species, monophyletic taxa are pools, or "packages," of genetic information. They are records of life's history; extant taxa at any one time simply represent the remaining subset of genetic information of any particular clade.

Thus taxa—always a prime focus of macroevolutionary theory, even when the *real* subject is adaptive transformation of organismic features—alone do not reveal the full story of evolutionary processes. Taxa are the result of evolutionary processes. But the actual "game of life" (the economic scene, the moment-by-moment *use* of economic adaptations and the consequences of such use in the economic organization of life) is not traditionally a subject matter of evolutionary theory. It is, rather, considered under the rubric of "ecology." But it is the action of organismic adaptations when put to use that determines the fates of their bearers, and the phylogenetic fate of the genetic information underlying the adaptations. The taxa of the genealogical hierarchy record success and continue to make surviving genetic information available; they are merely the ledger books, the fallout of history of economic systems up to the present moment. There is no "evolutionary process" distinct from the moment-by-moment economic processes of living—a subject to which we now turn.

Notes to Chapter 6

1. Reproductive tissues are generated anew from "somatic" tissue in plants; hence there is far less a clear-cut distinction between germ line and soma in plants than there is in animals.

2. It makes no difference whether reproductive or economic features are specified as synapomorphies in the systematics of higher taxa. Thus the placenta and presence of three middle ear bones are both characteristic of *placental mammals*.

3. The connection between heterochrony and the two separate classes of organismic phenotypic properties first arose in conversation with G. D. Edgecombe.

4. The history of classification of modes of heterochrony is summarized in Gould (1977). It is curious that most such classifications appear to have been assymmetrical: while paedomorphosis has apparently always been considered a matter of interplay of timing between aspects of somatic development and the onset of sexual maturation, no such coordinate definitions existed for "recapitulatory" phenomena. Indeed, Alberch et al. (1979) had to invent a term (*peramorphosis*) as a coordinate to *paedomorphosis*. McNamara (1986) may have been the first to present a wholly internally consistent classification of heterochronic phenomena, in which modes of peramorphosis are also seen to involve an interplay of timing between somatic and reproductive developmental timing.

5. Eldredge and Salthe (1984), however, point out that a species becomes extinct when reproduction is no longer possible. The dusky seaside sparrow (actually considered a distinct subspecies of *Ammodramus maritimus*) "officially" became extinct in 1987, when the last known individual (a male) died. But extinction had already occurred when the last sympatric female died, or when and if either of the last male and female living in close proximity could no longer reproduce.

6. It is curious, for just this reason, that Patterson and Smith (1987) report that very few of Sepkoski's paraphyletic fish and echinoderm families overlap the ranges of the more derived families; when they did find such overlap, Patterson and Smith (1987) did count the data as true extinctions.

7. For other examples of living fossils, plus additional discussion of the causal aspects of the phenomenon, see the compendium on "Living Fossils" edited by Eldredge and Stanley (1984).

Macroevolutionary Patterns II: Economic Systems

The reproductive activities of sexual organisms cause them to associate in small, local reproductive communities, or demes. All demes composed of organisms sharing an SMRS (Paterson, 1985) constitute a species. And because the SMRS of each species represents commonly held reproductive adaptations (shaped and maintained by sexual selection), and because such adaptive fertilization systems are therefore subject to further modification, new forms of SMRS develop from old forms, and speciation takes place as a matter of course. The ongoing process of speciation creates lineages of ancestral and descendant species, otherwise known as monophyletic taxa of higher rank.

The economic adaptations of organisms—the vast majority of organismic phenotypic attributes, and the focus of much of evolutionary theory—entail a wholly different set of consequences for organisms. Economic behavior results in (positive and negative) interactions with local organisms that share economic adaptations, ordinarily meaning simply conspecifics, but also potentially including local representatives of sibling species, or even of more remotely related taxa whose economic functions overlap to some significant degree (hummingbirds and nectar-feeding moths, for example, which are sometimes sympatric). Local economic groups of conspecific organisms are *avatars* (Chap. 5); avatars of many different species typically form the parts of local ecosystems.[1]

As briefly reviewed in Chap. 5, it is the moment-by-moment interactions among constituent, lower-level entities that supply the cohesion to each next higher level in the economic hierarchy. Like the genealogical hierarchy, the economic hierarchy consists of a list of ordered category terms, from more inclusive to less inclusive. Each item of like kind included within each of the levels is considered a spatiotemporally bounded entity (or "individual," sensu Ghiselin, 1974, see Eldredge, 1985). Thus, somatic cells interact to maintain tissue and organ cohesion, literally forming interactive parts of an organismic soma and keeping an organism together.[2] Similarly, sympatric conspecific organisms interact (cooperatively and/or competitively) to form local avatars; avatars interact to form cross-genealogical local ecosystems. And local ecosystems interact, and are thus bound together into more regional systems. The key aspect of such interactions is always energy flow (matter–energy transfer); the highest element of the economic hierarchy is the entire biosphere as it exists at any moment.

Damuth (1985) has argued that economic systems (especially his avatars) are not only interactors, but also "moremakers." Thus, in his view, economic entities fulfill both of Hull's criteria for selection (see p. 139), and elements of the economic hierarchy are all that actually need be considered in the *evolutionary* process. As we have already seen, and in stark contrast, evolutionary biologists have scarcely seen the need for including ecological entities in their considerations of the evolutionary process. Where interactive phenomena are considered at all (as in Dobzhansky's metaphor of adaptive peaks and ranges for species and higher taxa), elements of the genealogical hierarchy are considered to have interactive properties.

Can elements of the economic hierarchy be said to have genealogical (reproductive) properties? The answer is best approached by asking what the organization of nature would look like if organisms possessed *only* economic (matter–energy transfer) adaptations and lacked altogether reproductive adaptations (i.e., reproductive behaviors and functions). If organisms were only economic interactors, the answer seems reasonably clear that there would still be local associations of organisms sharing similar morphological and behavioral adaptations (largely, if not exclusively, conspecifics[3]), and such entities would interact in various ways to form local economic systems. The biotic world, in other words, would look and appear to act pretty much as it does anywhere at any given moment (except during breeding season!). In short, the hierarchical structure of economic systems appears to be a consequence strictly of the economic (interactive) activities of organisms.

Yet, as Damuth (1985) and others have observed, avatars and even local ecosystems occasionally do divide—producing two systems where there was once one. Superficially, this is a form of reproduction. But it is equally clear that, to be important in an *evolutionary* context, reproduction must have an effect on the fate of genetic information shared by a coherent genealogical entity. And ecosystems are patently cross-genealogical. The differential fates of elements of the ecological hierarchy do have an evolutionary impact, but only as their fates are recorded within demes, species, and monophyletic taxa (see below for more of the dynamics of cross-hierarchy interaction).

Yet, as already briefly discussed in Chap. 5, avatars and demes may, at least sometimes, be virtually one and the same entity. In such circumstances, in which a local entity of conspecifics is both a moremaker and an interactor, the possibility of "group selection" takes on reality.[4]

Thus it seems that the historical lack of consideration of ecological entities in evolutionary theory is understandable; because ecological entities lack a genealogical component, the relation of ecological entities to evolution is not immediately or intuitively obvious. Because evolutionary theory is mostly concerned with economic adaptations, though, ecological matters are clearly related *somehow* to the evolutionary process, though it is also quite clear that the connection does not lie in attributing economic attributes to genealogical entities.

Though ecological entities are not intrinsically historical entities in the way that species and monophyletic higher taxa are, nonetheless elements on the upper end of the scale of ecological entities have large-scale spatiotemporal distributions. Regional biotas are spread over large areas of continents, and over even larger areas of the oceanic regions of the world. And the fossil record shows that such systems are tolerably stable, remaining recognizably about the same, especially when compared with preceding and succeeding systems (see Olson, 1952). Regional marine biotal systems lasting as long as 10 million years are the norm in Paleozoic epeiric seas.

Miller (1986) has distinguished three basic levels of spatiotemporal distribution of cross-genealogical ecological systems (which he calls "communities"). For decades, paleontologists have sought, largely in vain, to apply the principles of *ecological succession* (through a series of two or more *seres*). The problem in making such observations reliably in the fossil record is one of temporal scale vs. mode of formation of fossil assemblages: as Miller (1986) points out (see Table 7.1), ecological succession takes place on a temporal scale on the order of 10 years, in general, far too quickly to be recorded in most depositional environments. Miller (1986), following earlier authors (e.g., Rollins, et al., 1979) proposed recognition of another process, *community replacement*, for a phenomenon much more readily observed by paleontologists (and often confused with true ecological succession). Community replacement, which Miller (1986) characterizes as taking place on a scale of from 10^2 to 10^6 years, involves the literal replacement of one community by another. The process is often, but not necessarily,

TABLE 7.1   Miller's Proposed Hierarchy of Community Temporal Dynamics of Soft-Bottom Marine and Estuarine Communities

Process	Preserved pattern	Estimated duration (years)*	Temporal dynamics involved
Community evolution	Community lineages	10^5 to 10^7 (?)	Origination and elaboration of new types of communities; community structural divergences; major biogeographical displacements and turnovers owing to extinctions: both species–environment and species–species interactions involved
Community replacement	Community sequences	10^2 to 10^6 (?)	Abrupt to gradual community transitions caused by environmental changes: long-period population–environment interactions predominate
Patch development	Amalgamated seres and/or pseudoseres	10 to 10^3 (?)	Prolonged occupation of seafloor area by benthic community undergoing many episodes of succession and/or response
Ecological succession	Seres	1 to 10	Autogenic, biotic changes in community composition and structure: short-term organism–organism interactions predominate
Community response	Pseudoseres	1 to 10	Allogenic, successionlike community changes; seasonal or cyclic short-term responses to environmental changes not leading to replacement: organism–environment interactions predominate
Community establishment	Noninteractive colonization sequences	10^{-3} to 10^{-1}	Earliest stages of substrate invasion in newly opened habitats; strongly dependent on availability and proclivity of colonizing larvae and motile adults: organism–environment interactions predominate

*"Durations are tentative estimates; processes differ in terms of temporal durations, predominant forcing factors, and the numbers and kinds of ecological units involved."
SOURCE: Miller, 1986, Table 1, p. 227.

abrupt (relative, that is, to the stability of the communities or ecosystems once established). In contrast to ecological succession, which functions largely as a response to biotic organizational factors, community replacement is seen as a direct response to environmental change, especially involving abiotic parameters.

Miller (1986) contrasts community replacement not only with ecological succession, but also with "community evolution," which involves development of new community types and "elaboration" of existing community types through the extinction of old, and the evolution of new, taxa. If we restrict the term "evolution" basically to the fate of genetically based information, evolution is probably best thought of strictly in connection with the genealogical hierarchy. Yet there is both continuity and change in overall community types on a grand scale (10^5 to 10^7 years), best seen through the perspective of higher taxic compositional stability and change, and "community evolution" is the term generally used for such phenomena. Bretsky (e.g., 1968, 1969) has been particularly incisive in analyzing ecological phenomena at the level of community evolution.

A key aspect to any notion of community evolution is the recognition of "analogous" ecological roles played by organisms of different monophyletic taxa over long periods of time. For example, from the Ordovician up at least through the end of the Paleozoic, nearshore marine communities tended to be dominated by mollusks. The mix of bivalve and gastropod taxa (nuculoid and pterioid bivalves and bellerophontid gastropods, among others) is repeated time and again, the world over. There are subdivisions of such communities correlated strongly with coarseness of the sedimentary substrate: large bellerophontids and large, epifaunal bivalves (plus homalonotid trilobites, nuculoid bivalves, and certain rhynchonellid brachiopods) recur repeatedly in silty and sandy substrates, while a more diverse assemblage of pleurotomarian gastropods and a greater mix of bivalves characterize more muddy environments. The point is, such community types are recognizable over truly prodigious spans of time, all the while with different taxa fulfilling the analogous ecological roles at different times.

This is the appropriate context for Dobzhansky's large-scale use of the adaptive landscape metaphor. Taxa—species and higher taxa—are not interactors. They do not have ecological niches or large-scale (taxic) analogues of niches, adaptive zones. Species and higher taxa are not parts of ecological systems—as Myers (1986), for example, has claimed. But organisms within species, hence within strings of genealogically linked species (i.e., higher taxa) *do* share genetically based economic adaptations. As we have already seen, species can be viewed as largely redundant packages of genetic information (i.e., when distributed as quasi-independent Wrightian "colonies"), with local organisms playing similar roles in a series of different local ecosystems. Higher taxa, on a grander scale, can be viewed in much the same way: felids as a family do not play a role of large spatiotemporal scale in some megaecological system. But cats play a variety of roles as carnivores in local ecosystems, and these roles have been repeated over and over at least since the Miocene in many ecosystems the world over. And similar roles can be played by organisms in other taxa, even those that appear catlike without being especially close relatives of cats (such as the extinct "saber tooths").

Thus ecological systems have histories, even though their primary organizational structure derives from moment-by-moment interactions. The ecological history of the biota is exactly analogous to human history, a sequence of events that owe their causation to the ongoing interactions of parts (in the case of human history, of humans, but also of larger-scale social systems, e.g., entire nation–states). It is not true evolution, but rather a complex result of past evolution and a cause of future evolution, as recorded in the genetic composition of organisms within species within higher taxa.

Eldredge (1985a, 1987; see also Brett et al., 1988 and in prep.) has briefly discussed a larger-scale version of Miller's (1986) "community replacement." Paleozoic regional epicontinental marine ecological systems typically persist on the order of 5 to 10 million years. For example, as Brett et al. (1988 and in prep.) have documented in detail, there are some 20 or so recognizable community types within the Hamilton group in New York State. The Hamilton seas occupied much of the eastern and central regions of North America for roughly 6 to 8 million years, waxing and waning, and in particular occasionally disappearing entirely in the central regions of the continent. Brett and colleagues recognize continual reappearance of community types in different areas within the Hamilton seas, the locus of communities depending upon sea level changes and (in the marginal seas of the east, particularly well studied in New York State), the westward encroachment of a complex deltaic sedimentary regime.

The point of the Hamilton situation is that while there are a large number of distinct community types, most of those communities remain recognizably the "same" throughout Hamilton time. The species found in the Hamilton seas in general persist, and for the most part display little change, throughout Hamilton time. (Not all Hamilton species by any means are found throughout the interval, but many of the most common species are present for the entire range of Hamilton time.) The critical issue then becomes: Do the community (ecosystem) "types" persist—and does the entire Hamilton economic system persist—because the species persist? Or do the species persist because the economic system persists? Or is it, somehow, both simultaneously? Cause and effect between origin, maintenance, and final disappearance of both economic systems and genealogical entities (taxa) is a complex issue and one that is central to a full understanding of macroevolution.

The Hamilton fauna and economic system begins and ends rather abruptly. Many of the Hamilton species belong to Old World province taxa: their closest relatives are found in slightly older rocks of present-day Europe (Rhine Valley) and northern Africa (e.g., Eldredge, 1972b; Bailey, 1983). The onset of the Hamilton fauna and economic system was triggered by the fusion of North America with Africa–Europe, a collision that caused the Caledonian orogeny and the beginning of deposition of terrigenous sediments in the eastern, downwarped marginal basin of North America. Prior to Hamilton times, carbonates were the primary constituent of the substrate.[5] Thus a profound physical change and a coordinate biogeographical recruitment were the ingredients of the abrupt change from the tropical carbonate seas of the Eifelian of North America ("Onondaga" and equivalents) to the muddy-bottom fauna of the eastern Hamilton seas. Carbonates occasionally formed during Hamilton times and are to be found especially in the interior epeiric seas. These, however, record a typically Hamilton fauna.

The termination of the Hamilton fauna some 6 to 8 million years after its appearance was likewise abrupt and records, also, physical environmental change. Enough of the derivation of the Hamilton ecosystem and biota has been sketched to show it to be an example, on a somewhat larger scale, of Miller's "replacement" phenomenon. The elements common to all such examples[6] are (1) extinction of a stable, well-established system through some physical agency—often interpretable as a single, if spatiotemporally large-scale, "event"—and (2) establishment of a succeeding system derived from surviving taxa, immigrant species, or some combination of both. The resemblance of the two systems depends on the similarity of the physical environments before and after the physical environmental "event" and the genealogical affinities of the taxa established in the succeeding ecosystem.

Vrba (1985) has examined such phenomena, concluding that most evolutionary change seems to occur in conjunction with cross-genealogical events, ecosystem turnovers in response to physical environmental events. She terms this the *turnover pulse hypothesis* and provides detailed examples from the later Tertiary environmental and especially mammalian taxic evolutionary history of Africa. In all such examples discussed so far in the literature, complex regional ecosystems are distributed over broad areas (entire sections of continental landmasses, for example—as in savannas of eastern and southern

Africa, or the marine epeiric seas covering the eastern and central regions of North America). There are many subdivisions of such broad regional systems, and these shift according to physical changes in the environment. During the history of any one of these large-scale economic systems, habitats shift but never completely disappear. There is some speciation, and some apparent extinction, but for the most part species persist (usually, but not necessarily, without accruing large amounts of economic adaptive change). Though there is no term for the ongoing speciation, Jablonski (e.g., 1986) refers to such patterns of extinction as "background"—as opposed to "mass" extinction, which characterizes the *ends* of such systems. Perhaps the term "background" (and possibly even "mass") applies as well to speciation phenomena during the course of history of these regional ecosystems ("background speciation"), and at the beginnings of some of them ("mass speciation").

That much of evolutionary change is restricted to speciation events—that economic adaptive change is causally connected with changes in reproductive adaptation (SMRS)—is not intuitively obvious; we have explored this connection at length in Chap. 4. The present proposition goes further: most economic adaptive change, and most speciation, seems to take place in definite *cross-genealogical* pulses. Though there is a sort of background, seemingly random[7] rate of speciation in geological time, most speciation events appear, like extinction events, to come in bunches—in cross-genealogical contexts (ecosystems)—as a response to the bunched cross-genealogical extinctions that have played a major and quite conspicuous role in the history of life.

Most discussions of large-scale adaptive change assume limitless time and uninterrupted histories of single lineages. Alternatively, as we have seen in earlier discussions, the old notion of *Stufenreihen*, in modern guise, might see speciation breaking up the smooth flow of transformation; and thus there may be an accumulation of species at various stages of the development of particular adaptations. In any case, complex adaptations (such as the morphology of "walking stick" insects) imply a great deal of relatively uninterrupted morphological transformation. Yet the context of adaptive change seems to be, in the largest sense, one in which extinction is unrelated to the particular adaptations of organisms. This is precisely the distinction Jablonski (1986) draws: Background extinction can be understood as the failure of adaptation, when environmental change outstrips organismic ability to track adaptively through natural selection. Mass extinction, in contrast, represents such significant and total environmental change that organisms in general, at least in many cases, simply cannot survive. Disappearance of an epeiric sea, or any other sweeping change in environment, amounts to elimination of habitat, and organisms disappear without respect to the precise nature of their adaptations.

We need now to examine in greater detail the general nature of interaction between components of the genealogical hierarchy (i.e., taxa) and elements of the economic hierarchy to pinpoint more precisely the patterns of causal interaction between the two.

The Evolutionary Plexus: Interactions Between Elements of the Genealogical and Ecological Hierarchies

The treatment of natural selection in earlier chapters represents, in essence, a return to Darwin's original conceptualization through the analytic device of Hull (1980), in which selection is seen as an interplay of *replicators* and *interactors*. The population genetics notion of *fitness*, or relative probability of reproductive success of an organism within a local population, elides into a single concept the dual nature of organisms both as ecological interactors and as reproducers (true replication being strictly located at the level of the genome). Thus causation in natural selection is obscured in the notion of fitness: the often tenuous (and certainly stochastic) relation between relative economic and relative reproductive success—the sine qua non of the shaping of economic adaptations through natural selection—is rendered more concrete, less uncertain, with the simple rubric of "relative fitness." Pulling the concepts of economic and reproductive functions apart permits a more careful assessment of the causal relation between the two. As we have already seen, Darwin (1859) manifestly understood the difference between the two and was (as many biologists following him have been) troubled by the loose connection between economic and reproductive success. One aspect of the problem (that there are *non*economic biases to reproductive success) led him directly to distinguish between *natural* selection, which pertain to economic adaptations, and *sexual* selection, which pertains to relative reproductive success as determined by variation strictly in aspects of reproductive physiology, morphology, and behavior.

Thus, from an evolutionary standpoint, the causal vector in natural selection (i.e., *not* sexual selection) runs *from* the economic interactor aspects of organisms *to* the reproductive: relative economic success governs relative reproductive success, and the latter amounts to a bias in the representation of genetic information in the succeeding generation.

But, as Mayr (e.g., 1964, p. xvi) and many other biologists have repeatedly said, (natural) selection is a "two-step process": the bias of economic success on reproductive success is the second step; the first is the production of variation within a local "population." What this means, translated into terms employed in this discussion so far, is that the reproductive behavior of organisms (1) maintains local economic populations of a species (avatars) and (2) (through various forms of mutation in the germ line, plus recombination, crossing over, and other molecular and cytogenetic events associated especially with sexual reproduction) presents a variable (nonuniform) spectrum of economic adaptations in that avatar. The ongoing impact of reproductive behavior on the composition of local avatars is just as profound as are the long-term effects of the economic activities of organisms in avatars on the genetic composition of demes, and therefore ultimately of species and monophyletic taxa.

Thus, reproduction produces, patently, an ongoing supply of organisms that are, for the greater parts of their lives, actors in the ecological arena. Relative success in the ecological arena in turn (and only in part) determines the proportions of preexisting genetic variation present in successive generations. This suggests that entities of the genealogical hierarchy (germ-line tissues and reproductive adaptations of organisms, demes, species, and monophyletic taxa) are (1) *passive* "ledger" books that record what has worked in the remote and more immediate past in terms of economic success, and (2) active suppliers of organisms to the economic arena, with all the attendant implications for the formation of larger-scale economic entities of the ecological hierarchy. Elements of the genealogical hierarchy are stable entities, i.e., stable configurations of genetic information. In terms of active process, then, the term "evolutionary process" is something of a misnomer: the active "work" (matter–energy transfer) of organic nature is largely subsumed in the economic hierarchy. The genealogical elements simply record genetic information and constantly resupply organisms to the ecological scene.

Once again, species emerge as a critical level. Both Dobzhansky (1937a, 1941) and Mayr (1942) stressed that *discontinuity* is a second aspect of evolution, coequal in importance with *diversity*. By "diversity," they meant the variety of apparent organismic phenotypic design in nature, adaptive in the main. By "discontinuity," they meant the partitioning of that diversity into discrete species (which they saw as reproductive communities). In Chap. 4, we reviewed recent theoretical work suggesting that speciation itself is causally implicated in the generation of that diversity. And speciation, moreover, is most certainly involved in the *preservation* of that morphological diversity, because speciation isolates the variation (otherwise susceptible to disappearance in local demes; see Futuyma, 1987), effectively injecting the diversity into the phylogenetic stream. It is the maintenance of that adaptively generated diversity that becomes critical when examining the role of species in the context of ecological–genealogical inter-hierarchical interactions.

As we have seen, species are not parts of ecosystems. Yet the role of species in the development and maintenance of ecosystems is critical. If we view species as composed of semiredundant packages of genetic information organized into semi-isolated demes (Wright's "semi-isolated colonies," see Dobzhansky, 1937*a*), the ecological importance of species becomes clear: Suitable habitats are continually colonized by organisms from adjacent demes. The phenomenon is recorded daily, even in the popular press. Thus, moose (*Alces alces*) have recently be-gun to become established in the Adirondack Mountains of New York State after an absence of roughly 100 years. Between roughly 1880 and 1980, moose in the Adirondacks were all transients. Reportedly, the recently established moose populations derive from several source areas, including New England and Canada. Clearly, moose living through the past 100 years in adjacent regions have remained eco-nomically and reproductively sufficiently similar to the avatars–demes of *A. alces* extirpated in the Adirondacks late in the past cen-tury to enable a "hybrid" fledgling population (actually, widely disseminated individual organisms currently numbering fewer than 100) to recognize appropriate habitat and resume moose exploitation of the Adirondack region.

Range changes of species in general reflect this phenomenon. Shrinking ranges, reflecting elimination of local avatars, represent as well local extinction of demes, and disappearance of genetic informa-tion. Range expansions represent recruitment to form new avatars, hence demes, and represent the spread of genetic information, in which new packages of largely redundant genetic information become established. Regional (geographic) differentiation has the effect of counteracting true, complete redundancy. According to some sources, the recent reestablishment of coyotes (*Canis latrans*) in eastern sec-tions of North America represents a spread eastward of some individ-uals from extant western populations. Those populations of coyotes, at least as presently constituted, consist of somewhat smaller organisms than the extinct "race" that formerly occupied the eastern regions.

In the marine realm, Johnson (1972) discusses an instance in which a sandbar slowly migrated across the floor of Tomales Bay (California), in places downgrading (to an earlier point of succession) and in others entirely obliterating the benthic community that had been in place. The benthic community was a patchwork of different stages of succession, all present side by side according to the recent physical history of the habitat. Recruitment of species locally elimi-nated came from elsewhere within the bay, or through larval dispersal from longer distances. Man-made ecological disasters (e.g., oil spills, nuclear accidents), natural disruptive events, and the appearance of new habitat space (as in the abrupt appearances of volcanic islands, e.g., Surtsey in 1963, or the completely made-over Krakatoa in 1883) have made the phenomenon of recruitment of avatars to (re-)form local ecosystems familiar.

As long as some part of a species remains extant, the possibility exists that a degraded or destroyed ecosystem will be reformed with pretty much the same cast of economic players (avatars). Thus the extinction of species looms as a crucial watershed in terms of ecosystem composition: as long as a single deme survives, the possibility that a species may be represented by avatars in a multiple system of habitats remains. Total extinction of a species, on the other hand, forever changes the spectrum of possible avatar composition of ecosystems.[8]

Thus extinction of species has strong implications for the complexion of future ecosystems. Ecosystems, of course, at any given moment are composed of the species that are extant and (geographically) available (historically occurring in a given region). That there are no bears in sub-Saharan Africa is more a reflection that bears, apparently, never have lived in sub-Saharan Africa than it is any reflection of their inability to occupy any of the current African habitats. But if a species becomes extinct, it is forever unavailable to stock any future ecosystem.

Thus it is tempting to suggest that it is the changes in species existence—speciation and extinction—that modify ecosystems through time. And, surely, speciation and Jablonski's background extinction do alter the complexion of local ecosystems through time. Yet, as we reviewed briefly earlier in this chapter, most biologists and paleontologists see extinction as a profoundly cross-genealogical affair. Mass extinction, whether regional or worldwide in scope, seems to a first approximation primarily an *economic*, rather than a genealogical, affair.

The search for causes of mass extinction (events in which many taxa become extinct in a relatively brief temporal interval, especially when compared with the prior longevity of the biotal system) is almost always in the direction of major disruption in one or more aspects of the physical environment. Extinctions are *measured* in terms of taxic extinction. Geographical extent is commonly correlated positively with taxonomic rank reached by the extinction event. As Raup and Sepkoski (e.g., 1982) have documented so well, the four largest extinctions known to have occurred in the Phanerozoic (roughly the last 600 million years) have been worldwide or nearly so in scope, have embraced both marine and terrestrial habitats, and by affecting *so many species* (up to 96 percent of extant species in the Permo-Triassic event; vide Raup, 1986*b*), have taken relatively more taxa of relatively higher rank than more regional extinctions are bound to account for.

Destruction of the Hamilton inland sea habitat, for example, eliminated perhaps as many as 300 species (i.e., of hard-shelled, fossilizable organisms), but far fewer genera, and perhaps not a single family. Sepkoski (1982) has, in contrast, documented the extinction of over 60 marine families (not all of which, presumably, are monophyletic) at the world-wide event near the end of the Devonian.

Extinction is a cumulative destruction of avatars in ecosystems; when extinction is sufficiently pervasive (in intensity, as well as areally), entire species become extinct; the more widespread the extinction event, the higher the average rank of the taxa that will disappear.

A survey of the putative causes of severe extinctions reveals a gamut from extraterrestrial impact—bolides of cometary or asteroidal origin (e.g., Alvarez et al., 1980; Raup, 1986a), possibly of a periodic occurrence according to Raup and Sepkoski, 1986—to climatic phenomena intrinsic to the several components of the earth's motion. All sophisticated causal explanations of widespread and large-scale extinction cite aspects (usually, if not necessarily, of the physical environment) that trigger the collapse of one or more large ecosystems. For example, both the spatial habitat shrinkage model of Newell (1967), Simberloff (1974), and Schopf (1974) and the impact scenario (Alvarez et al., 1980) explanations of mass extinction events cite a stepwise collapse of ecosystems stemming from the initial loss of ecologically key groups. Extraterrestrial impact itself, for example, is generally not held to have wiped out ecosystems in a single massive catastrophic event. Rather, the resultant cloud of particles suspended in the atmosphere is hypothesized to have occluded sufficient sunlight (for several years) to reduce photosynthesis drastically in land plants as well as in the marine phytoplankton. Virtually all explanatory models of mass extinction, then, share in common a reliance on stepwise (if sudden and dramatic) ecosystem collapse.

Major Diversity Changes Through Time

"Diversity" in traditional evolutionary discourse refers to the development of different phenotypes. Diversity in an ecological context means the number of different species (represented through avatars) present in a region, as in the comparison of diversity in the tropics and in the arctic tundra. Still another meaning of "diversity" is the number of species (as often measured through counts of higher taxa) present within a given monophyletic taxon through time.

Natural selection forms the basis of the causal explanation of phenotypic diversity. Controls of ecological diversity at various spatial and (particularly) temporal scales have been a major focus of ecological theory. Causes of changes in diversity within monophyletic taxa are even more difficult to establish than reasons for changes in ecological diversity are. Indeed, a major theme in modern macroevolutionary considerations of purely taxic diversity (measured as, say, genera within families) has been to establish that clade-diversity shapes (as depicted graphically in so-called spindle diagrams) can be distinguished from patterns generated "randomly" by an algorithm. Gould et al. (1987) have claimed that vectors of diversity change within clades yield far more "bottom heavy" spindle diagrams (i.e., in which diversity is concentrated during the early histories of clades) within early (Cambro-Ordovician) invertebrate clades than usually emerge in computer simulation studies. They conclude that there is a typical shape to the diversity of clades, one that can be interpreted as a unidirectional "vector of change" in evolution, though it is to be noted that many of the "real clades" examined by Gould et al. (1987) are paraphyletic or polyphyletic and thus are subject to the criticisms raised by Patterson and Smith (1987).[9]

We have briefly reviewed (Chap. 5) aspects of niche width in conjunction with a consideration of speciation rate controls (and the development and retention of adaptative change in speciation). The conclusion—that relative niche width is an important factor in determining both speciation and (species) extinction rates, as well as the development and rate of within-clade accumulation of adaptive change—again involves the control of economic (ecological) factors over genealogical phenomena. As Vrba (1988) has pointed out, there is no completely straightforward connection between aspects of the regulation of ecological diversity and within-clade diversity history, and care must be taken in attributing vicissitudes of clade-diversity composition to ecological causes. Yet, surely, clade-diversity patterns are primarily a means by which both nature and systematists can measure the effects of ecological events, both extinctions and subsequent diversifications, as well as longer periods of ecological status quo (with background extinction and speciation). The real action, the *cause* of diversity fluctuations no matter how measured, seems to reside firmly in the economic sphere, in elements of the ecological hierarchy.

Evolution is the fate—the stasis and change—of genetically based information. That information is stored in a nested series of entities: the genealogical hierarchy. But the determination of what genetic information (both the innovations and older information) is to be kept lies in the workings of the elements of the ecological hierarchy. To consider only the ledger-book results of the evolutionary process—the elements of the genealogical hierarchy—as most evolutionary biologists have done, is to miss the interactions of nature which spell out the moment-by-moment dynamics of life. Yet, to consider only the momentary cross-genealogical organization of life and ignore its organization into genealogical packages of genetic information is to miss the importance of the source of the information underlying the construction of that functional system. The notion of adaptation is the prime bridge between these two different organizational aspects of the biotic world. It now remains only to organize and summarize succinctly the major points in this book on the evolutionary development of adaptations: the evolutionary context of adaptive stasis and change.

Notes to Chapter 7

1. I will use the term "ecosystem" here; others might prefer to the term "community." "Ecosystem" generally includes the abiotic environment, as well as all the organisms in the system. "Community" refers exclusively to organisms living in association in a local area but suffers from the defect that very often, not all local organisms are included (as in the "avian community" of a given habitat). Because economic systems as envisioned here have a distinctly geographic aspect, inclusion of the abiotic realm in the entities composing the economic hierarchy is not seen as problematic.

2. In metazoan organisms, (mitotic) cell division, a holdover of reproductive processes, is equally important as cellular cohesion and interaction in maintaining the soma.

3. Without reproduction, there would be no species; hence the emphasis simply on shared (similar) economic adaptations. Further, without species, it is highly unlikely that economic adaptations would have achieved anything near the diversity and complexity true of the past 575 million years of biological history—hence the purely hypothetical nature of this thought experiment. Current ecological complexity is as fully dependent upon past episodes of speciation as the current complexion of genealogical systems is dependent upon the vicissitudes of economic systems.

4. As briefly noted in Chap. 5, Lloyd (1988), in fact, argues that when species are reduced to single demes or avatars, *species selection* itself becomes a real possibility. Though she concedes that it is only in such circumstances that species can be *interactors*, she concludes that species in general are interactors as well as moremakers, and thus that the objection to species selection based on the dual criteria of Hull (1980) is invalid. One interesting aspect of this particular debate is that species are most likely to consist of a single deme or avatar (1) in the earliest stages of their formation and (2) just before extinction (if extinction is through attrition and dwindling, rather than through a more catastrophic event).

5. The Needmore Shale of West Virginia records a muddy-bottom fauna of Onondaga (pre-Hamilton) age. The ecosystems are rather similar in aspect to those of the Hamilton, but the constituent taxa, insofar as they have been analyzed, are allied to the contemporaneous species elsewhere in the carbonate environments of North America. That the taxic elements of the Needmore did not play a more prominent role in the stocking of the Hamilton ecosystems (which appear to be dominated by Afro-European faunal elements) is interesting and not readily interpretable: the Needmore example shows that North American taxa were perfectly able to establish muddy-bottom ecosystems.

6. Brett and colleagues (1988 and in prep.) have discussed the natural division of the Paleozoic of North America into a number of "packages" of ecological systems. Each such package is comparable in spatiotemporal extent to the Hamilton ecological system.

7. The word "random" in evolutionary discourse generally carries the further connotation "with respect to a larger pattern or direction of change." Thus mutations are held to be "random," but only in the sense that they are unrelated to whatever regime of natural selection might obtain when the mutations occur. Mutations of a par-

ticular sort do not occur because the organism "needs" them. Otherwise mutations are definitely not random because they always have a definite physicochemical cause. Likewise for extinction: species, whether viewed within higher taxa or in the context of cross-genealogical systems may seem to appear and disappear "at random" because there is no overall, bunched pattern of extinction apparent. Yet there is always presumed to be a definite proximal cause for the extinction of any species.

8. The conservation movement has extensively debated the comparative wisdom of trying to preserve species vs. conserving entire habitat areas. Because species are crucial (once lost, their packaged genetic information is irretrievably gone), much of the conservation rhetoric in fact focuses on the need to save species. Yet many conservationists have realized that the real way to protect species is through the conservation of ecosystems, or, rather, large habitat areas that may embrace parts of a number of ecosystems. In that way, avatars will be conserved, and hence demes; and species represented within the area will automatically persist, regardless of the fates of avatars elsewhere (unless all members of one or more avatar(s) within the protected area are always recruited each generation from habitats outside the area, an unusual if not wholly impossible circumstance).

9. Kitchell and MacLeod (1988, p. 1192) have challenged the interpretation of Gould et al. (1987), arguing that the statistical value upon which Gould et al. (1987) based their conclusion "falls well within the expected distribution of clades generated by a purely random (time symmetric) branching process and hence is not significantly different from the expected shape of randomly branching (symmetrical) clades."

8

Summary
and
Conclusions

It is my intention, in this final chapter, to set out in abbreviated and coherent form the main points and arguments of the preceding chapters. The goal is to assess past theories of adaptation and their relation to ideas and models developed more recently.

The major premise of this book is that (neo-)Darwinian models of selection are indeed correctly identified as the essential ingredient of a theory of causal processes underlying both stasis and change in adaptation, but that the dearth of theory addressed to rates, degree, and timing of such change reveals the theory of adaptation to be incomplete.

The major set of ideas in the preceding chapters propounded to address these very issues centers on the distinction between *reproductive* and *economic* aspects of the organismic phenotype. "Reproductive" properties are all those phenotypic elements given over in whole or in part to reproductive functions; "economic" attributes are, consequently, all the rest, but are conceived of more positively as those features concerned with organismic "economics," obtaining and converting energy for processes of differentiation, growth, and maintenance of the organism itself. Because the two tend to behave at least partly independently, evolutionary patterns of both weak and strong covariation between the two are important ingredients of evolutionary theory.

The two classes are intricately interrelated, of course; in particular, energy and general somatic maintenance are clearly required for reproduction. Some phenotypic attributes have multiple functions, which may include some from each of the two categories. Also, phylogenetically, single-celled (especially prokaryotic) organisms show far less differentiation of structure and function along the lines of these two classes than metazoans (or even metaphytes) exhibit.

Nevertheless the two classes are tolerably distinguishable and, conceptually, when distinguished, provide keys to the understanding of the organization and workings of biological systems. In particular, several topics of concern to evolutionary theorists may be looked upon in rather a different light if the distinction between the two classes of organismic properties is kept firmly in mind. The following is a partial list of such topics—the final one on the biotic context of adaptive stasis and change serving as an introduction to a more detailed reiteration of key concepts associated with theories of macroevolutionary adaptive change.

A. Selection. It is a reasonable inference that most specifiable organismic phenotypic attributes are evolutionary adaptations, or at least "aptations" (Gould and Vrba, 1982). Hence there is a dichotomy in classes of adaptations corresponding to the two classes of phenotypic properties initially recognized. The first implication, then, is simply that *the two distinct kinds of selection originally recognized by Darwin—"natural" and "sexual"—correspond precisely to these classes.* Viewed this way, sexual selection is not simply a subset of natural selection. Nor is sexual selection simply mate selection, or to be considered only in conjunction with complexities of social behavior. Rather, it is present and affecting the reproductive anatomy, physiology, and behavior of all organisms. It is, as Darwin (1871, p. 256) originally defined it, "the advantage which certain individuals have over other individuals of the same sex and species, in exclusive relation to reproduction."

B. Interactors and replicators. The Hull-Dawkins distinction [broached at least in Hull's (1980) case as an analytic device to assess claims of selection above and below the organismic level] is isomorphic with the distinction between reproductive and economic classes of phenotypic attributes. It is only a slightly modernized version of Darwin's original vision to say that *natural selection is the statistical effect of relative economic success on relative reproductive success among conspecific organisms within a local population.* When natural selection is defined this way, conceptual difficulties with the term "fitness" are strikingly set off. Because Darwin and his intellectual descendants have realized the rather tenuous causal connection between economic and reproductive success, "fitness" has become a combinatorial term that glosses over the tenuous causal connection between economic and reproductive success, lending an air of determinism to (natural) selection that many biologists seem to prefer.

In contrast with natural selection, *sexual selection is relative reproductive success based solely on differential reproductive attributes.* These distinctions have further implications (as Hull originally intended they should have) for the assessment of selection at other levels.

C. Formation of stable entities at higher levels. When organisms simply *use* phenotypic attributes of either class, they find themselves as parts of larger systems that are formed as a direct consequence of that use. The two systems differ markedly—a difference that permeates the history of study of larger-scale biological systems. When reproductive attributes are in use, sexual organisms are parts of demes, and, perhaps more obviously, species. Species are stable entities held together by a shared *specific mate recognition system* (Paterson), i.e., the class of reproductive adaptations (formed and retained through sexual selection). Species form through the fragmentation of the SMRS through divergent sexual selection in allopatry.

Contra Mayr (e.g., 1982), species do not have niches; species perform no direct economic roles in natural systems. Because species speciate, i.e., make more of themselves, they are parts of monophyletic taxa and constitute an intermediate rung of what might be called a genealogical hierarchy (though see below).

The economic attributes of organisms likewise lead to associations of organisms into systems of a profoundly different nature from that of genealogical entities. Economic behavior in organisms leads to the existence of local *avatars* (Damuth, 1985)—interacting local populations of conspecifics that *do* have niches. (Avatars and demes may be, but usually are not, coextensive and thus may be, in a particular instance, "the same." This possibility has implications for higher-level selection; see below.) Avatars are locally associated cross-genealogically: it is the association of nonconspecifics into economic systems with energy flow that stems from organismic economic behavior. Local economic systems are loosely united into regionally ever-larger systems to form the functional "economic" hierarchy.

Put another way, as a consequence of having two sets of phenotypic properties (i.e., two sets of adaptations), organisms are simultaneously parts of two very different biotic systems. Most of the time, of course, it is the economic systems that are of importance.

D. Higher-level selection. It follows that *species selection* can only be an analogue of *sexual selection,* and not of *natural selection.* The SMRS can be viewed as a species-level property, thus removing the other major objection to species-selection models: the fact that most early discussions of species selection dealt with trends in economic organismic phenotypic properties.

Avatar selection is a reasonable higher-level analogue of natural selection if, and only if, avatars and demes are reasonably coincident. Ecosystems may fragment, but do not impinge coherently on genetically stored information; monophyletic taxa do not make more of themselves. Thus higher-level selection is not a valid issue with entities at these levels.

E. Heterochrony.   The prime link between ontogeny and phylogeny in terms of process theory, at least, lies in the realm of heterochrony. Most such theory is addressed to comparative patterns of development that contrast *onset of reproductive maturation with stages of development of economic attributes*. Thus the quasi-independence of the two classes of attributes within ontogeny is traditionally seen as giving rise to the marked differences between higher taxa.

F. Conflicting concepts of species.   The *genealogical* hierarchy, with its largest-scale categorical term of "monophyletic taxa," is related to, but not the same as, the *Linnaean* hierarchy. Cladists point out that the Linnaean hierarchy is also "genealogical." The problem exists, really, at the species level; recognition of stable reproductive communities with a shared SMRS (an evolutionist's species) contrasts strongly with the recognition of economically differentiated groups within such "biological" species. There will be a profound conflict, if it can be shown (on the basis of putative synapomorphy distribution) that some populations *within* an SMRS-defined species are actually more closely related to a second SMRS-defined species.

The situation is clarified with reference to the two classes of organismic properties. Genealogists use both economic and reproductive attributes to define monophyletic taxa: for example, three middle ear bones and placentas in mammals. Problems only arise when the economic attributes are more finely differentiated than the reproductive properties at the lowest levels of resolution. That is why botanists have traditionally balked at the Dobzhansky-Mayr *biological species concept*—precisely because economically differentiated taxa often hybridize (i.e., share an SMRS).

Thus at least the nature of the conflict between these two species concepts becomes clearer if we make the distinction in classes of organismic attributes. It could be argued that the Linnaean perspective is the older, and thus that the term "species" ought to be reserved as a taxon category just like "genus," "family," and so forth.

G. The biotic context of adaptive stasis and change. The distinction between classes of adaptation opens up possibilities of interplay between reproductive adaptive change (speciation, for the most part) and economic adaptive change. Such theory takes the form of triggers (facilitation; e.g., SMRS change as a goad for economic change) and conservors of change (e.g., Futuyma, 1987: speciation as a means of injecting economic adaptive change into the phylogenetic mainstream). Before summarizing such models, I will first simply list the major points latent in macroevolutionary theories of adaptive stasis and change.

1. There are two basic kinds of models of adaptive change, depending upon whether the "environment" (biotic, abiotic, or both) is considered to be changing, or not.

2. Since Wright (1932) presented his pictorial representation of the adaptive landscape, adaptive change is considered to occur either by shifts from one peak to another (where the peaks are either moving or stationary) or by the tracking of a moving adaptive peak, which may subsequently split to form two adaptive peaks. There is no single, consistent formulation of what an adaptive peak is; adaptive peaks are variously regarded as the equivalent of niches (or adaptive zones for large-scale taxa) or more precisely as relative fitness values. Dobzhansky (1951) presents the most familiar general model of adaptive change utilizing this imagery—in this model the entire diversity of life is explained with reference to the tracking of adaptive peaks through time.

3. Traditional, since Darwin, has been the tendency to expect rates of transformational change to vary somewhat, but to approximate regular, directional linearity. Because environments are constantly being modified, evolutionary change has generally been considered the norm, rather than the exception. The most recent manifestation of such imagery of nature underlies Van Valen's (1973) model of the Red Queen—in which a focal species must undergo constant evolutionary modification simply to remain extant, in the face of a constant degradation in the environment occasioned (in this particular model) by changes in other species with which the focal species is ecologically associated.

   Recently, a variety of biologists from different disciplines have incorporated the empirically well established notion of *stasis* into their considerations of patterns of adaptive change. Adaptive change seems in most instances to be concentrated in relatively brief episodes, preceded and followed by relatively much longer intervals of stability.

4. Simpson (1944) considered such patterns of change explicitly in terms of large-scale transformations. He argued that the apparently abrupt first occurrences of higher taxa in the fossil record implies relatively rapid rates of evolution, rather than missing intervals or simple nonpreservation of long skeins of intermediate forms. His earlier articulation of *quantum evolution* attempted to frame a theory of genetic processes suitable to explain the empirical patterns of the fossil record. In so doing, Simpson utilized Wright's imagery of the adaptive landscape, characterizing quantum evolution as relatively sudden shifts from one peak to another in the adaptive landscape.

5. Lande (e.g., 1986) and other geneticists recently have addressed Simpson's qualitative models in a quantitative fashion. At the heart of all such models is the consideration solely of the transformation of (implicitly *economic*) phenotypic properties.

6. Other attempts to model macroevolutionary transformation (e.g., Bock 1965, 1979), while also basically linearly transformational in outlook, have utilized the notion of *stable intermediate forms linked up to form "Stufenreihen."* Thus the Darwinian tradition still imagines relatively small steps accruing within episodes of large-scale phenotypic transformation, but such transformation may (1) be very rapid (yielding the appearance of saltation, e.g., in the fossil record) or (2) occur in a series of steps, e.g., as stable intermediate species. Saltational models (e.g., those of Goldschmidt, Schindewolf, and various more recent genetic and developmental formulations) in contrast consider at least the possibility of large-scale, single-step macroevolutionary change. This latter class of models is not pursued in any detail in this book.

7. Explanations for stasis (relative stability of phenotypic adaptive properties) generally emphasize *stabilizing selection.* Stabilizing selection is generally seen as an outcome of environmental stability; however, stasis can occur even in the face of environmental change by simple habitat tracking. Habitat rearrangement is the normal outcome of environmental change, and stasis results so long as organisms "recognize" and continue to exploit familiar habitat.

Wright (e.g., 1932), as part of his *shifting balance theory,* developed a picture of species distributed into a number of semi-isolated "colonies" (later known as *demes*). Because the adaptive (and genetic drift) histories of each of these local populations are likely to be different from those of conspecific populations integrated into other ecosystems, we should expect no single, concerted directional pattern of adaptive change to occur specieswide. Rather, oscillations of a basic pattern of geographical variation—

stasis—should be the usual pattern to emerge if Wright's picture of species structure is an accurate description of nature. As a corollary, the Red Queen should hold only for local populations within ecosystems and not serve as a descriptor for specieswide phylogenetic histories. Moreover, patterns of directional change recorded in the fossil record should hold for local populations and not for species as a whole.

8. The major innovation of the modern synthesis (i.e., in my opinion) was Dobzhansky's (1937*a*) and Mayr's (1942) addition of the concept of *discontinuity* to the concept of the generation of (adaptive, phenotypic) *diversity*. Dobzhansky and Mayr changed the emphasis in the concept of *species* from a collectivity of similar organisms (that could also interbreed) to a community of interbreeding organisms (that also tended to resemble one another closely).

Because natural selection generates a continuum of adaptive diversity, Dobzhansky and Mayr argued in general that reproductive discontinuity must underlie discontinuities in general phenotypic (adaptive, generally "economic") organismic features. Through time, species lineages continued to be divided up into subsegments, according to the older criteria of phenotypic resemblance.

New reproductive communities (new species) were generally held to arise in allopatry through the simple accumulation of adaptive change, generally economic, but also conceivably reproductive per se (the two classes of property were not, of course, explicitly distinguished). Thus economic divergence underlies reproductive divergence initially, but the discontinuity in reproductive adaptation imposes discontinuity in general phenotypic properties.

9. The theory of *punctuated equilibria* (Eldredge and Gould, 1972) sees species as reproductive communities with beginnings, histories, and terminations. Stasis within species facilitates recognition and argues against the model that species can be divided into chronologically successive lineage segments.

Eldredge and Gould (1972) moreover take the causal argument a step further, maintaining that *adaptive change in general only occurs in conjunction with speciation, i.e., the development of reproductive discontinuities.* In light of the distinction between economic and reproductive attributes as outlined in this book, this is to say that *economic change is unlikely to accrue to any significant degree without reproductive change.*

10. Paterson's (1985 and earlier references) concept of SMRSs makes the distinction between reproductive and economic organismic attributes explicit with respect to species and speciation. According

to Paterson, new species arise by changes in the species-specific mate recognition system; such changes are under the control of selection for continued mate recognition in allopatry. Moreover, such selection is obviously *sexual* selection, and most of the time, mate recognition entails *stabilizing sexual selection* as opposed to brief episodes of *directional sexual selection,* during which aspects of the SMRS are modified.

11. In principle, reproductive and economic adaptive change are independent. In empirical reality, patterns of stasis and change indicate that while some change in both systems might occur without concomitant change in the other, there is an assymmetrical relation such that reproductive discontinuity (change in reproductive adaptations) may occur without significant economic adaptive change (as seen in sibling species), but that little or no economic change can occur unless and until there is reproductive adaptive change (i.e., speciation). *Speciation is hypothesized to be necessary, but not sufficient, for significant economic adaptive change to occur.*

12. There are a number of possible causal pathways that explain this pattern, falling into two basic categories: speciation (SMRS change) may act (1) to conserve economic adaptive diversity and (2) to actually trigger or promote such economic adaptive change.

13. Speciation acts as a conserver of adaptive change. Darwin, in some contexts, spoke of species as "permanent varieties." Wright's picture of species distributed as a series of semiautonomous local populations also emphasizes the ephemeral nature of most within-species variation. Most demes become extinct, or are reintegrated with other demes. With SMRS change, unique economic attributes become established in separate stable entities ("species") with their "own separate evolutionary role(s) and tendencies"—as Simpson (1961, p. 153) put it as part of his very definition of "evolutionary species."

It is further argued that newly formed reproductive communities (newly formed species) have a greater probability of survival if they are ecologically differentiated somewhat from the ancestral species. Economically less well differentiated species are likely simply to be swamped by the more numerous members of the parental species. Thus there is bias towards the accrual of economically differentiated species. Moreover, survival of new species is higher in stenotopes because they are ecologically more disjunct, on average, than are eurytopes. Thus higher rates of speciation in stenopic lineages is a reflection more of survival of fledgling species than of a higher intrinsic rate of SMRS disruption in stenotopes over eurytopes. However, on a long-term basis, eurytopes have lower extinction rates than stenotopes.

14. Speciation acts as an inducer of economic adaptive change. It is further argued that SMRS disruption (speciation) can trigger further economic adaptive change, particularly in populations near the periphery (therefore edaphic extremes) of the ancestral species range.

15. Macroevolutionary patterns include trends, adaptive radiations, arrested evolution, and steady state (the accumulation of little or no interspecific economic adaptive change).

    Trends record directional transformation of one or more aspects of economic adaptive features. Though some "trends" actually represent misreadings of historical data, nonetheless patterns of directional transformation in phylogenetic history are real enough. Formerly, the (neo-)Darwinian model of directional selection working to transform properties within species was generally extrapolated to yield patterns of among-species directional change. However, such explanations conflict with observations of stasis interrupted by occasional episodes of change, and with the interpretation that significant economic change occurs and accrues mostly in conjunction with true speciation.

16. Species as spatiotemporally bounded entities ("individuals") can be sorted through biases in birth and/or extinction rates within higher taxa (monophyletic *clades*). Such sorting contributes to the generation of macroevolutionary patterns, including trends.

17. *Sorting* of species may result either from lower-level causation (i.e., causation arising from properties of organisms themselves—Vrba's [e.g., 1980] *effect hypothesis*) or from *species selection*. Neither the effect hypothesis nor species selection is a hypothesis bearing on the generation of adaptations per se: organismic phenotypic adaptations are shaped by natural and sexual selection. Rather, organismic phenotypic properties are distributed within species; through the differential histories of species, distributions of phenotypic properties form patterns (such as trends) through phylogenetic time.

18. Because species arise from the reproductive behaviors of organisms, and because such reproductive communities are not parts of specifiable economic systems, species themselves are seen as parts of a genealogical hierarchy and not as members of the ecological hierarchy. Moreover, "species selection" is analogous with "sexual selection," and not with "natural selection," which requires economic interaction along with reproductive behavior to operate (see item D above). Because the SMRS is a species-level property,

species selection is a real possibility; however, the connection between species selection and the distribution of organismic economic properties (patterns of which, e.g., "trends," first prompted the hypothesis) is weak, and entails concepts such as *hitchhiking*.

19. Because economic and reproductive attributes of organisms lead to the existence of two hierarchical systems in which organisms are simultaneously members, evolution in general is the result of interactions between the two systems. The connection is most clearly seen in the causal process of natural section itself. In general, the genealogical hierarchy consists of stable entities (germline genome, reproductive properties of organisms, demes, species, monophyletic taxa) that (1) supply the genetically based information (players) to the ecological arena and (2) record the differential results, the "outcome," from the economic side. It is with the economic elements (economic aspects of organisms, avatars, local and regional ecosystems), held together by dynamic interactions among subparts, that the game of life is largely played.

20. Complex adaptations, then, are imagined to accrue through a series of stable intermediates (forming *Stufenreihen*). *Stufenreihen,* however, may not be as internally wholly unidirectional as often depicted. *The stable intermediates forming stages of Stufenreihen are held to be species, in the strict Mayr-Dobzhansky-Paterson sense.*

21. Mass extinctions are cross-genealogical and occur without regard for the stage of accrual of complex adaptations within single lineages. Mass extinctions commonly eliminate complex adaptations and reset the ecological, hence evolutionary, clock. Thus, without mass extinctions, more elaborately complex adaptations would likely accrue, but, on the other hand, truly novel adaptations—the sort that mark large-scale taxic differences, and the usual stuff of "macroevolution"—would be correspondingly even more rare in phylogenetic history than they appear to have been.

References

Alberch, P., S. J. Gould, G. F. Oster, and D. B. Wake. 1979. Size and shape in ontogeny and phylogeny. *Paleobiology* 5:296–317.

Altokhov, Y. P. 1982. Biochemical population genetics and speciation. *Evolution* 36:1168–1181.

Alvarez, L. W., W. Alvarez, F. Asaro, and H. V. Michel. 1980. Extraterrestrial cause for the Cretaceous-Tertiary extinction. *Science* 208:1095–1108.

Arnold, A. J., and K. Fristrup. 1982. The theory of evolution by natural selection: A hierarchical expansion. *Paleobiology* 8:113–129.

Bailey, J. B. 1983. Middle Devonian Bivalvia from the Solsville Member (Marcellus Formation), central New York State. *Bull. Amer. Mus. Nat. Hist.* 174:193–326.

Barton, N. H., and B. Charlesworth. 1984. Genetic revolutions, founder effects, and speciation. *Ann. Rev. Ecol. Syst.* 15:133–164.

Bock, W. J. 1965. The role of adaptive mechanisms in the origin of higher levels of organization. *Syst. Zool.* 14:272–287.

Bock, W. J. 1970. Microevolutionary sequences as a fundamental concept in macroevolutionary models. *Evolution* 24:704–722.

Bock, W. J. 1972. Species interactions and macroevolution. *Evol. Biol.* 5:1–24.

Bock, W. J. 1979. The synthetic explanation of macroevolutionary change—a reductionistic approach. *In* J. H. Schwartz and H. B. Rollins (eds.), *Models and Methodologies in Evolutionary Theory. Bull. Carnegie Mus. Nat. Hist.* 13:20–69.

Bock, W. J. 1986. Species concepts, speciation and macroevolution. *In* K. Iwatsuki, P. H. Raven, and W. J. Bock (eds.), *Modern Aspects of Species*, pp. 31–57. University of Tokyo Press, Tokyo.

Bretsky, P. W. 1968. Evolution of Paleozoic marine invertebrate communities. *Science* 159:1231–1233.

Bretsky, P. W. 1969. Evolution of Paleozoic benthic marine invertebrate communities. *Palaeogr. Palaeoclimatol. Palaeoecol.* 6:45–59.

Brett, C. E., and K. D. Miller. 1988. Hierarchical scales of paleoecological processes in a muddy epeiric sea. *SEPM Mid-Yr. Mtg Abstr.*, 5:8.

Brett, C. E., K. D. Miller, and G. C. Baird. In prep. A temporal hierarchy of paleoecological processes within a Middle Devonian epeiric sea. *In* Miller III, W., *Paleont. Soc. Spec. Pub.*

Brooks, D. R., and E. O. Wiley. 1986. *Evolution as Entropy. Toward a Unified Theory of Biology.* University of Chicago Press, Chicago.

Brown, W. L., and E. O. Wilson. 1956. Character displacement. *Syst. Zool.* 5:49–64.

Bush, G. L. 1975. Modes of animal speciation. *Ann. Rev. Ecol. Syst.* 6:339–364.

Carson, H. L. 1982. Speciation as a major reorganization of polygenic balances. *In* Barigozzi, C. (ed.), *Mechanisms of Speciation*, pp. 411–433. Alan R. Liss, New York.

Coope, G. R. 1979. Late Cenozoic fossil Coleoptera: Evolution, biogeography and ecology. *Ann. Rev. Ecol. Syst.* 10:247–267.

Cracraft, J. 1986. The origin and early diversification of birds. *Paleobiology* 12:383–399.

Cracraft, J. 1987. Species concepts and the ontology of evolution. *Biol. Phil.* 2:329–346.

Cracraft, J. 1988 (ms.). Species as entities of biological theory. *In* Ruse, M. (ed.), *What the Philosophy of Biology Is.* Elsevier, Amsterdam.

Damuth, J. 1985. Selection among "species": A formulation in terms of natural functional units. *Evolution* 39:1132–1146.

Darwin, C. 1859. *On the Origin of Species.* John Murray, London.

Darwin, C. 1871. *The Descent of Man, and Selection in Relation to Sex.* John Murray, London.

Darwin, 1872. *On the Origin of Species.* 6th ed. John Murray, London.

Dawkins, R. 1976. *The Selfish Gene.* Oxford University Press, New York and Oxford.

Dawkins, R. 1986. *The Blind Watchmaker.* W. W. Norton, New York and London.

De Beer, G. R. 1954. *Archaeopteryx lithographica.* British Museum (Natural History), London.

Delson, E., and A. L. Rosenberger. 1984. Are there any anthropoid primate living fossils? *In* N. Eldredge, and S. M. Stanley (eds.), *Living Fossils.* Springer-Verlag, New York.

Dobzhansky, T. 1937a. *Genetics and the Origin of Species.* Reprint ed., 1982. Columbia University Press, New York.

Dobzhansky, T. 1937b. Genetic nature of species differences. *Amer. Naturalist* 71:404–420.

Dobzhansky, T. 1941. *Genetics and the Origin of Species.* 2nd ed. Columbia University Press, New York.

Dobzhansky, T. 1951. *Genetics and the Origin of Species.* 3rd ed. Columbia University Press, New York.

Donoghue, M. J. 1985. A critique of the biological species concept and recommendations for a phylogenetic alternative. *Bryologist* 88:172–181.

Dover, G. A. 1982. Molecular drive: A cohesive mode of species formation. *Nature* 299:111–117.

Eldredge, N. 1971. The allopatric model and phylogeny in Paleozoic invertebrates. *Evolution* 25:156–167.

Eldredge, N. 1972a. Systematics and evolution of *Phacops rana* (Green, 1832) and *Phacops iowensis* Delo, 1935 (Trilobita) from the Middle Devonian of North America. *Bull. Amer. Mus. Nat. Hist.* 147:45–114.

Eldredge, N. 1972b. Notes on the trilobites of the Hamilton group of the Chenango Valley region. *N. Y. State Geological Assoc. Guidebook,* 44th Ann. Mtg., F19–F24.

Eldredge, N. 1976. Differential evolutionary rates: Some comments on Schopf et al. *Paleobiology* 2:174–177.

Eldredge, N. 1979. Alternative approaches to evolutionary theory. *In* J. H. Schwartz and H. B. Rollins (eds.), *Models and Methodologies in Evolutionary Theory. Bull. Carnegie Mus. Nat. Hist.* 13:7–19.

Eldredge, N. 1982. *The Monkey Business: A Scientist Looks at Creationism.* Washington Square Press (Pocket Books), New York.

Eldredge, N. 1984. Simpson's inverse: Bradytely and the phenomenon of living fossils. *In* N. Eldredge and S. M. Stanley (eds.), *Living Fossils,* pp. 272–277. Springer-Verlag, New York.

Eldredge, N. 1985a. *Unfinished Synthesis. Biological Hierarchies and Modern Evolutionary Thought.* Oxford University Press, New York.

Eldredge, N. 1985b. *Time Frames.* Simon and Schuster, New York.

Eldredge, N. 1986. Information, economics and evolution. *Ann. Rev. Ecol. Syst.* 17:351–369.

Eldredge, N. 1987. *Life Pulse.* Facts On File, New York.

Eldredge, N., and J. Cracraft. 1980. *Phylogenetic Patterns and the Evolutionary Process. Method and Theory in Comparative Biology.* Columbia University Press, New York.

Eldredge, N., and S. J. Gould. 1972. Punctuated equilibria: An alternative to phyletic gradualism. *In* T. J. M. Schopf (ed.), *Models in Paleobiology,* pp. 82–115. Freeman, Cooper, San Francisco.

Eldredge, N., and S. J. Gould. 1974. Reply to Hecht. *Evol. Biol.* 7:303–308.

Eldredge, N., and M. J. Novacek. 1985. Systematics and paleobiology. *Paleobiology* 11:65–74.

Eldredge, N., and S. N. Salthe. 1984. Hierarchy and evolution. *Oxford Survs. Evol. Biol.* 1:182–206.

Eldredge, N., and S. M. Stanley (eds.). 1984. *Living Fossils.* Springer-Verlag, New York.

Eldredge, N., and I. Tattersall. 1982. *The Myths of Human Evolution.* Columbia University Press, New York.

Endler, J. A. 1986. *Natural Selection in the Wild. Monogrs. in Pop. Biol.* 21. Princeton University Press, Princeton.

Farris, J. S. 1977. On the phenetic approach to vertebrate classification. *In* M. K. Hecht, P. C. Goody, and B. M. Hecht (eds.), *Major Patterns in Vertebrate Evolution,* pp. 823–850. Plenum, New York.

Fisher, D. C. 1984. The Xiphosurida: Archetypes of bradytely? *In* N. Eldredge and S. M. Stanley (eds.), *Living Fossils,* pp. 196–213. Springer-Verlag, New York.

Fortey, R. A., and R. P. S. Jefferies. 1982. Fossils and phylogeny—a compromise approach. *In* K. A. Joysey and A. E. Friday (eds.), *Problems of Phylogenetic Reconstruction. Syst. Assoc. Spec.* 21:197–234. Academic Press, London.

Fox, L. R., and P. A. Morrow. 1981. Specialization: Species property or local phenomenon? *Science* 211:887–893.

Fryer, G., and T. D. Iles. 1969. Alternative routes to evolutionary success as exhibited by African cichlid fishes of the genus *Tilapia* and the species flocks of the great lakes. *Evolution* 23:359–369.

Futuyma, D. J. 1987. On the role of species in anagenesis. *Amer. Naturalist* 130:465–473.

Ghiselin, M. T. 1974. A radical solution to the species problem. *Syst. Zool.* 23:536–544.

Ghiselin, M. T. 1987. Species concepts, individuality, and objectivity. *Biol. Phil.* 2:127–143.

Gingerich, P. D. 1974. Stratigraphic record of Early Eocene *Hyopsodus* and the geometry of mammalian phylogeny. *Nature* 248:107–109.

Gingerich, P. D. 1976. Paleontology and phylogeny: Patterns of evolution at the species level in Early Tertiary mammals. *Amer. J. Sci.* 276:1–28.

Goldschmidt, R. 1940. *The Material Basis of Evolution.* Yale University Press, New Haven.

Gould, S. J. 1977. *Ontogeny and Phylogeny.* Harvard University Press, Cambridge.

Gould, S. J. 1980*a.* Is a new and general theory of evolution emerging? *Paleobiology* 6:119–130.

Gould, S. J. 1980*b.* G. G. Simpson, paleontology, and the modern synthesis. *In* E. Mayr and W. B. Provine (eds.), *The Evolutionary Synthesis: Perspectives on the Unification of Biology,* pp. 153–172. Harvard University Press, Cambridge.

Gould, S. J. 1988. Trends as changes in variance: A new slant on progress and directionality in evolution. *J. Paleont.* 62:319–329.

Gould, S. J., and N. Eldredge. 1977. Punctuated equilibria: The tempo and mode of evolution reconsidered. *Paleobiology* 3:115–151.

Gould, S. J., N. L. Gilinsky, and R. Z. German. 1987. Asymmetry of lineages and the direction of evolutionary time. *Science* 236:1437–1441.

Gould, S. J., and E. S. Vrba. 1982. Exaptation—a missing term in the science of form. *Paleobiology* 8:4–15.

Greenacre, M. J., and E. S. Vrba. 1984. A correspondence analysis of biological census data. *Ecology* 65:984–997.

Haacke, W. 1893. *Gestaltung und Vererbung.* Weigel, Leipzig.

Hallam, A. 1976. Stratigraphic distribution and ecology of European Jurassic bivalves. *Lethaia* 9:245–259.

Hennig, W. 1950. *Grundzüge einer Theorie der phylogenetischen Systematik.* Deutscher Zentralverlag, Berlin.

Hennig, W. 1965. Phylogenetic systematics. *Ann. Rev. Entomol.* 10:97–116.

Hennig, W. 1966. *Phylogenetic Systematics.* University of Illinois Press, Urbana.

Hull, D. L. 1973. *Darwin and His Critics.* Harvard University Press, Cambridge.

Hull, D. L. 1976. Are species really individuals? *Syst. Zool.* 25:174–191.

Hull, D. L. 1978. A matter of individuality. *Phil. Sci.* 45:335–360.

Hull, D. L. 1980. Individuality and selection. *Ann. Rev. Ecol. Syst.* **11**:311–332.

Huxley, J. S. 1942. *Evolution: The Modern Synthesis.* Harper, New York.

Huxley, J. S. 1958. Evolutionary processes and taxonomy with special reference to grades. *Uppsala Univ. Arssk.* **1958**:21–38.

Jablonski, D. 1986. Background and mass extinctions: The alteration of macroevolutionary regimes. *Science* **231**:129–133.

Jablonski, D. 1987. Heritability at the species level: Analysis of geographic ranges of Cretaceous mollusks. *Science* **238**:360–363.

Johnson, R. G. 1972. Conceptual models of benthic marine communities. *In* T. J. M. Schopf (ed.), *Models in Paleobiology*, pp. 148–159. Freeman, Cooper, San Francisco.

Kitchell, J., and N. MacLeod. 1988. Macroevolutionary interpretations of symmetry and synchroneity in the fossil record. *Science* **240**:1190–1193.

Lande, R. 1976. Natural selection and random genetic drift in phenotype evolution. *Evolution* **30**:314–334.

Lande, R. 1979. Quantitative genetic analysis of multivariate evolution, applied to brain: body size allometry. *Evolution* **33**:402–416.

Lande, R. 1985. Expected time for random genetic drift of a population between stable phenotypic rates. *Proc. Natl. Acad. Sci.* **82**:7641–7645.

Lande, R. 1986. The dynamics of peak shifts and the pattern of morphological evolution. *Paleobiology* **12**:343–354.

Levinton, J. 1988. *Genetics, Paleontology and Macroevolution.* Cambridge University Press, Cambridge and New York.

Levinton, J. S., and C. M. Simon. 1980. A critique of the punctuated equilibria model and implications for the detection of speciation in the fossil record. *Syst. Zool.* **29**:130–142.

Lewis, H. 1966. Speciation in flowering plants. *Science* **152**:167–172.

Linnaeus, C. 1758. *Systema naturae.* 10th ed. Stockholm.

Lloyd, E. A. 1988. *The Structure and Confirmation of Evolutionary Theory.* Praeger (Greenwood Press).

MacFadden, B. J. 1976. Cladistic analysis of primitive equids, with notes on other perissodactyls. *Syst. Zool.* **25**:1–14.

Malmgren, B. A., W. A. Berggren, and G. P. Lohmann. 1983. Evidence for punctuated gradualism in the Late Neogene *Globorotalia tumida* lineage of planktonic foraminifera. *Paleobiology* **9**:377–389.

Margulis, L. 1974. Five-kingdom classification and the origin and evolution of cells. *Evol. Biol.* **7**:45–78.

Maynard Smith, J. 1987. Darwinism stays unpunctured. *Nature* **330**:516.

Mayr, E. 1942. *Systematics and the Origin of Species.* Reprint ed., 1982. Columbia University Press, New York.

Mayr, E. 1954. Change of genetic environment and evolution. *In* J. Huxley, A. C. Hardy, and E. B. Ford (eds.), *Evolution as a Process*, pp. 157–180. Allen & Unwin, London.

Mayr, E. 1964. Introduction to reprint edition of Darwin (1859), *On the Origin of Species*, pp. vii–xxvii. Harvard University Press, Cambridge.

Mayr, E. 1969. *Principles of Systematic Zoology.* McGraw-Hill, New York.

Mayr, E. 1974. Cladistic analysis or cladistic classification? *Z. Zool. Syst. Evol.-forsch.* **12**:94–128.

Mayr, E. 1980. Biographical essays. G. G. Simpson. *In* E. Mayr and W. B. Provine (eds.), *The Evolutionary Synthesis*, pp. 452–463. Harvard University Press, Cambridge.

Mayr, E. 1982*a*. *The Growth of Biological Thought.* Harvard University Press, Cambridge.

Mayr, E. 1982*b*. Speciation and macroevolution. *Evolution* **36**:1119–1132.

Mayr, E. 1988. The species category. Essay 19 of Mayr, E., *Toward a New Philosophy of Biology*, pp. 315–334 (essay first published 1986). Harvard University Press, Cambridge.

Mayr, E., E. G. Linsley, and R. L. Usinger, 1953. *Methods and Principles of Systematic Zoology.* McGraw-Hill, New York.

Mayr, E., and W. B. Provine (eds). 1980. *The Evolutionary Synthesis: Perspectives on the Unification of Biology.* Harvard University Press, Cambridge.

McCune, A. R. 1982. On the fallacy of constant extinction rates. *Evolution* 36:610–614.

McNamara, K. J. 1986. A guide to the nomenclature of heterochrony. *J. Paleont.* 60:4–13.

Miller III, W. 1986. Paleoecology of benthic community replacement. *Lethaia* 19:225–231.

Mishler, B. D., and R. N. Brandon. 1987. Individuality, pluralism, and the phylogenetic species concept. *Biol. Phil.* 2:397–414.

Morton, J. E. 1958. *Molluscs.* Hutchinson & Co., London.

Myers, N. 1986. Tackling mass extinction of species: A great creative challenge. *The Horace M. Albright Lectureship in Conservation,* XXVI:1–40. University of California, College of Natural Resources, Berkeley.

Nelson, G. J. 1970. Outline of a theory of comparative biology. *Syst. Zool.* 19:373–384.

Nelson, G. J., and N. I. Platnick. 1981. *Systematics and Biogeography. Cladistics and Vicariance.* Columbia University Press, New York.

Newell, N. D. 1967. Revolutions in the history of life. *Geol. Soc. Amer. Spec. Paper* 89:63–91.

Newman, C. M., J. E. Cohen, and C. Kipnis. 1985. Neo-darwinian evolution implies punctuated equilibria. *Nature* 315:400–401.

Novacek, M. 1984. Evolutionary stasis in the elephant-shrew, *Rhynchocyon. In* N. Eldredge and S. M. Stanley (eds.), *Living Fossils.* Springer-Verlag, New York.

Olson, E. C. 1952. The evolution of a Permian vertebrate chronofauna. *Evolution* 6:181–196.

Ostrom, J. H. 1979. Bird flight: How did it begin? *Amer. Sci.* 67:46–56.

Paterson, H. E. H. 1985. The recognition concept of species. *In* E. S. Vrba (ed.), *Species and Speciation. Transvaal Mus. Monogr.* 4:21–29.

Patterson, C. 1977. The contribution of paleontology to teleostean phylogeny. *In* M. K. Hecht, P. C. Goody, and B. M. Hecht (eds.), *Major Patterns in Vertebrate Evolution,* pp. 579–643. Plenum, New York.

Patterson, C., and A. B. Smith. 1987. Is the periodicity of extinctions a taxonomic artefact? *Nature* 330:248–251.

Platnick, N. I., and H. D. Cameron. 1977. Cladistic methods in textual, linguistic, and phylogenetic analysis. *Syst. Zool.* 26:380–385.

Provine, W. B. 1989. Progress in evolution and meaning in life. *In* Nitecki, M. (ed.), *Evolutionary Progress,* pp. 49–74. University of Chicago Press, Chicago.

Raup, D. M. 1986a. *The Nemesis Affair.* W. W. Norton, New York.

Raup, D. M. 1986b. Biological extinction in earth history. *Science* 231:1528–1533.

Raup, D. M., and J. J. Sepkoski, Jr. 1982. Mass extinctions in the marine fossil record. *Science* 215:1501–1503.

Raup, D. M., and J. J. Sepkoski, Jr. 1986. Periodic extinction of families and genera. *Science* 231:833–836.

Rensch, B. 1947. *Neuere Probleme der Abstammungslehre.* F. Enke, Stuttgart.

Rensch, B. 1960. *Evolution Above the Species Level.* Columbia University Press, New York.

Rollins, H. B., M. Carothers, and J. Donahue. 1979. Transgression, regression, and fossil community succession. *Lethaia* 12:89–104.

Ryan, M. J., and W. Wilczynski. 1988. Coevolution of sender and receiver: Effect on local mate preference in cricket frogs. *Science* 240:1786–1788.

Schaeffer, B. 1948. The origin of a mammalian ordinal character. *Evolution* 2:164–175.

Schaeffer, B., M. K. Hecht, and N. Eldredge. 1972. Phylogeny and paleontology. *Evol. Biol.* 6:31–46.

Schaefer, S. A., and G. V. Lauder. 1986. Historical transformation of functional design: Evolutionary morphology of feeding mechanisms of loricarioid catfishes. *Syst. Zool.* 35:489–508.

Schindewolf, O. H. 1950. *Grundfragen der Palaontologie.* Schweizerbart, Stuttgart.

Schoch, R. M. 1986. *Phylogeny Reconstruction in Paleontology.* Van Nostrand Reinhold, New York.

Schopf, T. J. M. 1974. Permo-Triassic extinctions: Relation to sea-floor spreading. *J. Geology* 82:129–143.

Schopf, T. J. M. 1984. Rates of evolution and the notion of living fossils. *Ann. Rev. Ecol. Syst.* 12:245–292.

Schwartz, J. H. 1987. *The Red Ape.* Houghton Mifflin, Boston.

Sepkoski, Jr., J. J. 1982. *Compendium of Fossil Marine Families. Contr. Biol. Geol. Milwaukee Publ. Mus.* 51:1–125.

Sepkoski, Jr., J. J. 1987. Reply to Patterson and Smith. *Nature* 330:251–252.

Sheldon, P. R. 1987. Parallel gradualistic evolution of Ordovician trilobites. *Nature* 330:561–563.

Simberloff, D. S. 1974. Permo-Triassic extinctions: Effects of area on biotic equilibrium. *J. Geology* 82:267–274.

Simpson, G. G. 1944. *Tempo and Mode in Evolution.* Columbia University Press, New York.

Simpson, G. G. 1945. The principles of classification and a classification of the Mammalia. *Bull. Amer. Mus. Nat. Hist.* 85:1–350.

Simpson, G. G. 1953. *The Major Features of Evolution.* Columbia University Press, New York.

Simpson, G. G. 1959a. The nature and origin of supraspecific taxa. *Cold Spring Harbor Symp. Quant. Biol.* 24:255–271.

Simpson, G. G. 1959b. Mesozoic mammals and the polyphyletic origin of mammals. *Evolution* 13:405–414.

Simpson, G. G. 1961. *Principles of Animal Taxonomy.* Columbia University Press, New York.

Simpson, G. G. 1963. The meaning of taxonomic statements. *In* S. L. Washburn (ed.), *Classification and Human Evolution,* pp. 1–31. Aldine, Chicago.

Simpson, G. G. 1970. Uniformitarianism. An inquiry into principle, theory, and method in geohistory and biohistory. *In* M. K. Hecht and W. C. Steere (eds.), *Essays in Evolution and Genetics in Honor of Theodosius Dobzhansky,* pp. 43–96. Appleton-Century-Crofts, New York.

Simpson, G. G. 1975. Recent advances in methods of phylogenetic inference. *In* W. P. Luckett and F. S. Szalay (eds.), *Phylogeny of the Primates, a Multidisciplinary Approach,* pp. 3–19. Plenum, New York.

Sokal, R. R., and T. J. Crovello. 1970. The biological species concept: A critical evaluation. *Amer. Naturalist.* 104:127–153.

Stanley, S. M. 1975. A theory of evolution above the species level. *Proc. Natl. Acad. Sci.* 72:646–650.

Stanley, S. M. 1979. *Macroevolution: Pattern and Process.* W. H. Freeman, San Francisco.

Stanley, S. M. 1984. Does bradytely exist? *In* N. Eldredge and S. M. Stanley (eds.), *Living Fossils,* pp. 278–280. Springer-Verlag, New York.

Stanley, S. M. 1985. Rates of evolution. *Paleobiology* 11:13–26.

Stanley, S. M. 1986. Population size, extinction, and speciation: The fission effect in Neogene Bivalvia. *Paleobiology* 12:89–110.

Stanley, S. M., and X. Yang. 1987. Approximate evolutionary stasis for bivalve morphology over millions of years: A multivariate, multilineage study. *Paleobiology* 13:113–139.

Stenseth, N. C., and J. Maynard Smith. 1984. Coevolution in ecosystems: Red Queen evolution or stasis? *Evolution* 38:870–880.

Stringer, C. B., and P. Andrews. 1988. Genetic and fossil evidence for the origin of modern humans. *Science* 239:1263–1268.

Tattersall, I. 1986. Species recognition in human paleontology. *J. Human Evol.* 15:165–175.

Templeton, A. R. 1981. Mechanisms of speciation—a population genetic approach. *Ann. Rev. Biol. Syst.* 12:23–48.

Thompson, P. 1983. Tempo and mode in evolution: Punctuated equilibrium and the modern synthetic theory. *Phil. Sci.* 50:432–452.

Tiegs, O. W., and S. M. Manton. 1958. The evolution of the Arthropoda. *Biol. Revs.* 33:255–337.

Van Valen, L. 1973. A new evolutionary law. *Evol. Theory* 1:1–30.

Van Valen, L. 1976. Energy and evolution. *Evol. Theory* 1:179–229.

Vrba, E. S. 1980. Evolution, species and fossils: How does life evolve? *S. Afr. J. Sci.* 76:61–84.

Vrba, E. S. 1984a. What is species selection? *Syst. Zool.* 33:318–328.

Vrba, E. S. 1984b. Evolutionary pattern and process in the sister-group Alcelaphini-Aepycerotini (Mammalia:Bovidae). *In* N. Eldredge and S. M. Stanley (eds.), *Living Fossils*, pp. 62–79. Springer-Verlag, New York.

Vrba, E. S. 1985. Environment and evolution: Alternative causes of the temporal distribution of evolutionary events. *S. Afr. J. Sci.* 81:229–236.

Vrba, E. S. 1988 (ms.). Ecological predictions for macroevolutionary patterns in the fossil record. *In* N. C. Stenseth (ed.), *Coevolution in Ecosystems and the Red Queen Hypothesis*. Cambridge University Press, Cambridge.

Vrba, E. S., and N. Eldredge. 1984. Individuals, hierarchies and processes: towards a more complete evolutionary theory. *Paleobiology* 10:146–171.

Vrba, E. S., and S. J. Gould. 1986. The hierarchical expansion of sorting and selection: Sorting and selection cannot be equated. *Paleobiology* 12:217–228.

Westoll, T. S. 1949. On the evolution of the Dipnoi. *In* G. L. Jepsen, G. G. Simpson, and E. Mayr (eds.), *Genetics, Paleontology and Evolution*, pp. 121–184. Princeton University Press, Princeton.

Whewell, W. 1837. *History of the Inductive Sciences*. Parker, London.

White, M. J. D. 1968. *Modes of Speciation*. W. H. Freeman, San Francisco.

Wiley, E. O. 1981. *Phylogenetics: The Theory and Practice of Phylogenetic Systematics*. John Wiley, New York.

Williams, G. C. 1966. *Adaptation and Natural Selection. A Critique of Some Current Evolutionary Thought*. Princeton University Press, Princeton.

Williamson, P. G. 1981. Paleontological documentation of speciation in Cenozoic molluscs from Turkana Basin. *Nature* 293:437–443.

Wolpoff, M., X. Z. Wu, and A. Thorne. 1984. Modern *Homo sapiens* origins: A general theory of hominid evolution involving the fossil evidence from East Asia. *In* F. H. Smith and F. Spencer (eds.), *The Origin of Modern Humans: A World Survey of the Fossil Evidence*. Alan R. Liss, New York.

Wright, S. 1931. Evolution in Mendelian populations. *Genetics* 16:97–159.

Wright, S. 1932. The roles of mutation, inbreeding, crossbreeding, and selection in evolution. *Proc. Sixth Int. Congr. Genetics* 1:356–366.

Wright, S. 1945. *Tempo and Mode in Evolution:* A critical review. *Ecology* 26:415–419.

Wright, S. 1982. Character change, speciation, and the higher taxa. *Evolution* 36:427–443.

Wright, S. 1988. Surfaces of selective value revisited. *Am. Nat.* 131:115–123.

INDEX